M000236606

CHOOSING

HAPPY

44 PROVEN HACKS TO DEFEAT SADNESS AND EMBRACE A JOY FILLED LIFE

HEIDI FARRELLY

COPYRIGHT © 2018, HEIDI FARRELLY

ALL RIGHTS RESERVED. NO PART OF THIS PUBLICATION MAY BE REPRODUCED, STORED IN A RETRIEVAL SYSTEM, OR TRANSMITTED IN ANY FORM OR BY ANY MEANS, ELECTRONIC, MECHANICAL, PHOTOCOPYING, RECORDING, OR OTHERWISE, WITHOUT THE PRIOR WRITTEN PERMISSION BY THE PUBLISHER.

ISBN: 9780994517166

EDITED BY ELAINE ROUGHTON
EMAIL: H.ELAINE.ROUGHTON@GMAIL.COM

COVER ART BY SILLIER THAN SALLY DESIGNS
WEBSITE: WWW.SILLIERTHANSALLY.COM

THIS BOOK IS DEDICATED TO MY SISTER-FRIENDS. THOSE AMAZING PEOPLE WHO GIVE UNCONDITIONAL LOVE AND SUPPORT IN TOUGH TIMES — WITHOUT JUDGEMENT.

FOR MICHELLE, THANK YOU FOR SHOWING ME THE WAY, AND CONTINUING TO DO SO FOR OTHERS.

FOR VANESSA, WHOSE STRENGTH AND COURAGE UNDER PRESSURE INSPIRE ME.

AND FOR LAUREN, WHO HELD MY HOPE WHEN I COULDN'T HOLD IT MYSELF, AND WHO CONTINUES TO ENCOURAGE AND UPLIFT ME.

I WOULDN'T BE WHERE I AM NOW WITHOUT YOU ALL.

XX ♥ XX

INTERNAL ARTWORKS BY:

4LIE_ARTWORKS
ASHWIN PILLAI
ASYLE
BEN DAVID PUGH
CAROLINE RUSS
COLLETTE PLANT
COLOURDAZE
CRAIG DAWSON
CRISTIAN YAPUR 'CRIYADRAW'
JAMES CRUMBO
JEN FONTANILLA
JOSE JAIMES
KAROLINA OWCZAREK

KELLY EDELMAN
KELSEY NICOLE ASKEW
LILY BOWDLER
LISAMCGRUERART
LUCKY DAVINCITY
MARINA MARKOVA 'M.M.'
MJ.OANNE
RACHEL 'WOLVES'
SAMANTHA OLIVIA SWAT
VANESSA EVETTS
YEREDI FERNANDEZ LARA
'HARPAW'

FOR MORE INFORMATION ON THESE AMAZING ARTISTS PLEASE VISIT
WWW.HOW2WITHOUT.COM

THIS BOOK HAS BEEN WRITTEN TO PROVIDE COPING MECHANISMS AND TO BRING CHANGE TO THOSE WHO FIND THEY ARE SAD, OVERWHELMED, IRRITABLE, OR LETHARGIC ON A REGULAR BASIS. ITS AIM IS TO BOOST DAILY HAPPINESS, AND TEACH METHODS YOU CAN USE TO DIMINISH ANXIETY, SADNESS, NEGATIVE THINKING, AND APATHY.

CHOOSING HAPPY IS NOT A GUIDE FOR THOSE WITH DEPRESSION, NOR IS IT MEANT TO REPLACE THERAPY OR MEDICATION. I STRONGLY ENCOURAGE YOU TO SEEK IMMEDIATE MEDICAL HELP IF YOU ARE HAVING ANY FEELINGS OF SUICIDE OR SELF—HARM.

INSTEAD, *CHOOSING HAPPY* IS ALL ABOUT STAYING HEALTHY MENTALLY. BECAUSE MENTAL HEALTH IS NOT JUST ABOUT HEALTH CONDITIONS SUCH AS DEPRESSION AND ANXIETY. INSTEAD IT IS ABOUT WELLNESS. THE WORLD HEALTH ORGANISATION DESCRIBES MENTAL HEALTH AS:

"A STATE OF WELL—BEING IN WHICH EVERY INDIVIDUAL REALISES HIS OR HER OWN POTENTIAL, CAN COPE WITH THE NORMAL STRESSES OF LIFE, CAN WORK PRODUCTIVELY AND FRUITFULLY, AND IS ABLE TO MAKE A CONTRIBUTION TO HER OR HIS COMMUNITY."

AND THIS IS WHAT I WANT FOR YOU. TO BE WHOLE AND HAPPY. BODY, MIND, AND SPIRIT.

TABLE OF CONTENTS

INTRODUCTION
♪♫♪ DANCING ON MY OWN — TIESTO REMIX ♪♫♪

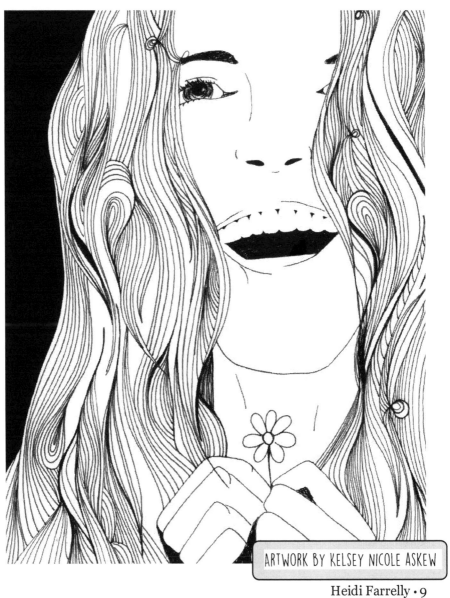

ARTWORK BY KELSEY NICOLE ASKEW

Scientists now believe as little as 10% of our total happiness is influenced by our circumstances. Another 50% is determined by our genes. So, what influences the remaining 40%? We do. Us. Numero Uno. *We personally influence 40% of our own happiness.* And that is huge! That means that no matter what is going on in your life, or what genes you possess, you have the ability to increase your happiness by 40%.

You see, happiness can be learned. It doesn't just magically appear, as many people seem to think. It isn't something we receive, or something we are entitled to. Rather, it's something we have to prioritize, and work towards. We have to actively strive to be happy. We have to search for it, create it, and choose it.

Being happy is a conscious decision.

We are the only ones responsible for our own happiness. Past circumstances, family, friends, jobs, environment, they all impact our lives on one level or another, but they don't control them. Not unless we allow them to. Only you can make the decision to be happy. But it is one of the most powerful decisions you can make.

Just because happiness is a personal choice doesn't mean it's easy, though. Many people have no idea how to start choosing happiness, and if you don't know how to fight low mood, it's almost impossible to win. It's like fighting a mugger when you're blindfolded, wielding only a feather. It's not that you should give up fighting. You just need to gain clarity and get some better weapons!

And that's what *Choosing Happy* is all about.

Its proven hacks will help you combat the sadness and apathy, the self-loathing, negativity, and irritability. It will enable you to push through the layers of sadness that have overlaid your life, and help you embrace daily joy.

With depression affecting 350 million people worldwide, it's becoming increasingly important to address low mood BEFORE it cripples you. If you often feel sad or low, then this book is for you. If you simply want to bring more happiness and unadulterated joy into your life, then this book is also for you. Are you tired? Cranky? Do you find it hard to get excited about anything? Then this book is definitely for you.

There is a vast difference between depression and low mood, and yet they are intrinsically linked. Think of depression like a raging storm. Sometimes there are warning signs of its arrival if you know what to look for (although sometimes there aren't). If you suspect you're bracing for a storm or if you're entering the calm after it, then this book is for you.

If, however, you are in the middle of that raging storm, then this book is *not* for you. It will be. Hopefully soon. But right now, you need more than these life hacks to help you through the craziness that is depression.

You will need to take more aggressive measures such as a combination of therapy and medication. Please, please seek help, even if you're not sure whether you have depression or not. Sometimes it's hard to recognise depression until after the fact. Tell a friend, family member, talk to your doctor, TELL SOMEONE, as you can't do this alone. They will all help you weather the storm and eventually find your way out.

Statistics show that only a third of depression sufferers worldwide seek help. And yet 80-90% of people with depression respond well to treatment, and almost all patients gain some relief from their symptoms. Please see the appendix for a full list of websites, hotlines, symptoms, and warning signs that you can use to assess yourself and seek help where needed.

There are many reasons people have low mood, and sadness. Sometimes it appears quickly, but often it is the combination of many things over an extended period of time: Stress, lack of sleep, anxiety, loss, loneliness, hereditary factors, ill health, or past experiences can all contribute. Each person is different. I don't know what led you to experience it, but I do know I can help you defeat it.

What makes me so certain? Because several years ago, I was where you are now. I was sad without really having a reason. I was cranky and irritable pretty much all the time. I felt guilty for yelling at my child, constantly seeing only the bad things in life, and generally being a crappy human being, but I couldn't seem to stop doing it!

My husband told me I seemed to be sad from the minute I woke up, until the minute I went to bed. And he gave me an ultimatum: Be happier or go and talk to someone. And by "someone" he meant one of those freaky head shrinking people...

It took his insight to really make me 'see' how bad it had gotten. And that was the moment. Right there. That was the moment I decided I was going to be happy. Whatever it took.

I started researching depression and working out what made me tick. I found ways to head my bouts of sadness off at the pass, to make sure I focused on my responses to different situations and how I reacted to them. And I used any hacks I could to make sure each day, I was choosing happiness over sadness. And slowly but surely, I got better.

All the hacks I walk you through in *Choosing Happy* have been proven to help people struggling with low mood. Many of them I have personally used, with great success, and still use today. Not all of them will work for every person, but at least some of them will work for you. Be open minded. Experiment. Persevere. Take what works for you and discard the rest.

I am a bestselling finance author (money, for goodness' sake, not mental health), but I wrote *Choosing Happy* because I wanted to give people something that I didn't have two years ago: A simple, easy-to-follow guide to choosing happiness and overcoming low mood, instead of the boring, weighty tomes that I kept wading through!

My finance books are known for being easy to read, even though they're packed with info, and *Choosing Happy* is no different. It's written in everyday language, and it's already helping people get their lives back on track.

Low mood *is* beatable! You do *not* have to live your life in a fog of negativity. And I, for one, am not going to let sadness be my constant companion.

I choose to live an outrageously happy life. What about you?

CHOOSING HAPPY HOW TO
♪♫♪ GOOD LIFE – ONEREPUBLIC ♪♫♪

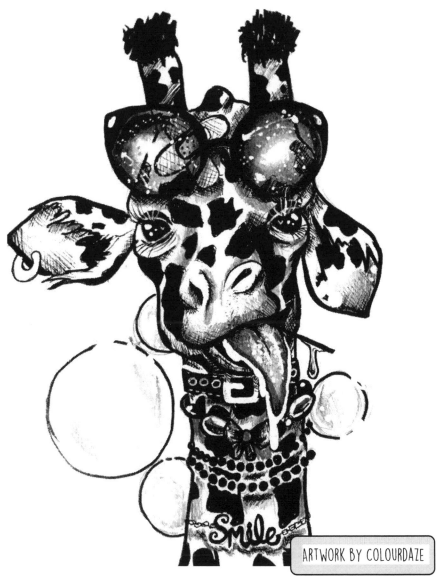

ARTWORK BY COLOURDAZE

Choosing Happy has been designed to be read pretty much however you like. You can open it at random and read the boxed facts, quotes, or bolded text. You can read it solidly from cover to cover, or you can simply enjoy the fantastic illustrations.

Choosing Happy is separated into sections which deal with different areas of your body, mind, and life. Within each of these sections are several chapters which, while all written on a similar topic, are standalone.

This means you can read one chapter, one section, or the whole book. It's entirely up to you. Kind of like "Choose Your Own Adventure" books, only you won't find yourself stuck in quicksand with no escape. I promise. (P.S. Don't read chapter 36 if you don't want to end up in quicksand.)

Each chapter is laid out to include as much information as possible, in the easiest and least confusing way. Here's what you get in a chapter:

Music ♫ ♪ Every chapter starts with the title and artist of a song that either reflects the sentiments of the chapter or is simply a feel-good tune. Look it up! Music is amazing for buoying flagging spirits and getting you grooving! I've also put together five albums on Spotify with happy songs in different genres. Follow me (heidifarrelly), steal the songs to create your own playlists, or suggest more with the hashtag #choosinghappyplaylist on Facebook, Instagram, or Twitter.

Quote 📝 You've got to love a good quote. Some people know just what to say, and when to say it. So, I've stolen their awesomeness and put at least one in each chapter for you to enjoy. You can thank me later.

Story 📖 This is the text, the words, the information. Kinda need this.

Science ☢ I love facts, but not everyone does! With this in mind I have put all the scientific facts (otherwise known as gibberish) into boxes. This means you can read them or skip them. Entirely up to you.

Illustrations ✐ There is a hand-drawn illustration to go with each chapter of *Choosing Happy*. If all you're feeling up to is flicking through the book and looking at pictures, then you're going to love these! They've come from a diverse range of talented artists, and you can find more info on each one and their work on my website www.how2without.com. Enjoy!

Further Study ▶ Sometimes I touch on a subject that, while it's interesting, is not talked about in depth in *Choosing Happy*. If this happens, you'll see the play symbol ▶ next to the subject. You can find links to books, articles, and videos related to these topics on my website, www.how2without.com which will give you more information - if you're interested.

Linked to 🔗 No, that's not LinkedIn. If you see the little chain symbol, it means that something we just talked about is also covered in another chapter, usually in more depth. If you're interested in knowing more straight away, then head on over. Otherwise, just read it when you get there.

Recap ⤸ No chapter would be complete without a wrap up of everything we've been over. This is especially helpful if you don't feel up to reading an entire chapter. You can simply flick to the end and read the recap for a basic understanding of what was covered.

Action steps ✎. And last but not least - some homework. Don't worry, you don't have to recite a list of all the planets.

(Don't forget Pluto is no longer classified as a planet. There'll be a pop quiz in chapter 36. It's the only way to get out of the quicksand.)

Instead, the 'homework' consists of actionable steps that you can take to get the hack we've just covered working for you. They are broken down into three stages: '**Do Now,**' '**Plan to Do,**' and '**Work Towards.**'

As you can see, each chapter packs a big punch. But you will never feel overwhelmed or swamped, because you can read as little or as much as you like. This means you can take it at your own speed while still moving towards a happier you.

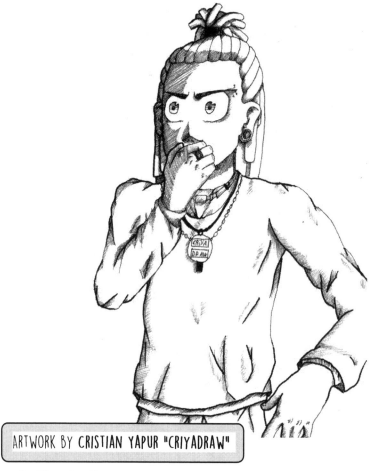

ARTWORK BY CRISTIAN YAPUR "CRIYADRAW"

LESSONS IN LOW MOOD
♪♫♪ STRONGER (WHAT DOESN'T KILL YOU) — KELLY CLARKSON
♪♫♪

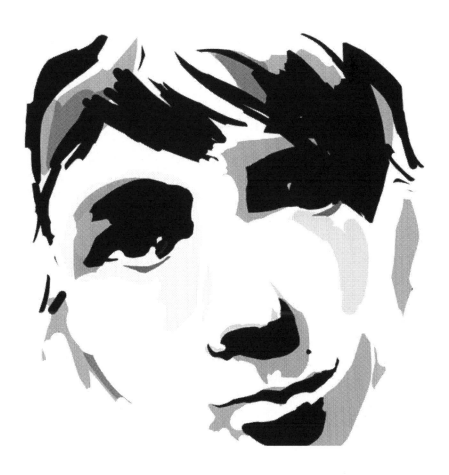

ARTWORK BY COLLETTE PLANT

So, what is low mood? Well, let's start with what it's not. It's not depression. Depression is a serious mental illness that needs a combination of therapy and medication to recover from. Unlike depression, low mood can be improved by taking positive action and resolving issues that may be causing it.

Low mood is also not a figment of your imagination, or something that you can just snap out of if you only tried harder. It is used to describe feelings of sadness, apathy, and a lack of enjoyment in your life. It also encompasses things you might not expect, like irritability, changes in your sleep patterns or appetite, and tiredness.

Low mood overstays its welcome like an annoying guest you just can't get rid of. It overshadows your life and makes you feel hopeless about your future. It affects your memory, your concentration, and sets up a constant stream of negativity inside your brain. All these things ensure you never see, or appreciate, the good things happening around you.

These are all symptoms of low mood▶. It's not all just tears and apathy (although there's plenty of this too). Low mood can wear many disguises, and sadly, too many of us seem to be struggling with it, not just occasionally, but every day. And yet there seems to be a great deal of confusion surrounding low mood. People who have never experienced long stretches of sadness find it hard to see how much it can affect your day-to-day life.

I like to describe it to people as a headache you've had for weeks. It doesn't matter what you do, you can't shake it. Things like pain medication may numb it, and there are times when it even disappears, but you know it's still lurking, waiting to come roaring back. You get so used to coping with the headache, and living your life with its restrictions, you start to think it's normal. But it is anything but normal!

I know life sucks sometimes. There are usually patches where it sucks a lot! But when we've been 'down' for an extended period of time, I think we forget how to focus on and choose those things that make us happy. We forget to try. Because being happy doesn't necessarily come as naturally and as spontaneously as people make out. You have to strive for it, search for it, recognize it for what it is, and grab it with both hands when you find it.

Everyone knows and experiences sadness on some level, throughout their lives. And this is a good thing! We need sadness to process the tough times in our lives, to help us grieve, and to be the flip side of our happiness coin.

Have you seen the kids movie 'Inside Out?' SPOILER ALERT! At the end of the movie you find out that we need all our emotions in life to create a well-rounded human being. This means no one emotion should dominate. Happiness, anger, fear, and sadness too. We need them all! Your emotions make you who you are and allow you to experience every aspect of life. Sadness is not a bad thing.

Until it is.

When sadness lingers, when it starts to eat into our psyche, when it becomes overwhelming, or a 'normal' part of our lives, then sadness is no longer part of our emotional repertoire, but the sum total of it. Sadness in this form can be debilitating, exhausting, and can block the normal happiness of life out.

One of the biggest steps you can take when combating a problem is to acknowledge one exists. Denial is a slippery slope, and you cannot start to heal until you face your issues head on. The day I acknowledged that my sadness and irritability was a real issue, and not just tiredness, or me being a horrible person, was the day I started to get better.

"Mental health is not a personal failure, in fact, if there is failure, it is to be found in the way we have responded to people with mental and brain disorders."
-DR. GRO HARLEM BRUNTLAND, DIRECTOR GENERAL OF WHO-

Sometimes, acknowledging there's something wrong is the hardest part. I grew up in New Zealand, and Kiwis don't really talk about emotional things. We only hug if we haven't seen each other in ages, or if something really exciting happens, or if someone is upset. And even then, it can be awkward. In fact, we tend to shy away from emotional displays in general (unless it's to do with rugby - and then we're pretty emotional)!

So, admitting I had a problem to myself, and opening up to others about it, was one of the hardest things I've ever done. Mental health still has a huge stigma, not just in New Zealand, but in almost every country in the world, and can be seen as a weakness or a failing in an individual. People worry others will see them as 'soft,' 'crazy,' or 'just lazy,' and this outdated way of thinking is preventing people from getting the help they need.

Many people think that they are alone in their feelings of sadness and low mood, but you couldn't be more wrong. Millions of people worldwide suffer with mood disorders. You probably know someone who is struggling, even if you don't realise it.

You think you're the only one who keeps your emotions hidden? Many people with sadness and low mood don't let others know what's going on when they're behind closed doors. They feel ashamed, don't want to burden their friends and family, and don't think others can help anyway.

Please, tell people when there is something wrong. Don't just think it will go away on its own, because generally it doesn't. And your friends and family want to be there for you. They want to help. But they're also not mind readers. It doesn't matter if you only confide in one person at first. Just tell someone. You will be amazed at how good it feels. If you don't feel comfortable telling them in person, text them. You can always catch up later on, face to face.

People may not understand what you're struggling with, but they will understand you need help, and most are happy to offer it. And sometimes that's all that matters. Low mood is an issue you share with many other people around the globe, so don't be surprised if you find out that the people you do talk to have already had experience with low mood.

When I first opened up about my depression, I was surprised by how many of my friends and family were suffering along with me. They'd tell me that they'd been going through the same thing, or they knew someone who was, and suddenly it wasn't such a scary thing to talk about after all. ✐1

In speaking up to help myself, I received a double whammy of good. I not only realised I wasn't suffering alone, I was also able to help others open up, and that felt pretty awesome too.

Low mood is no different from that headache we talked about earlier. Most of us have had headaches at some point in our lives. We have no problem talking about them to others, seeking advice, trying different methods for treating them naturally, or simply taking medication for them. Essentially, you do everything in your power to get rid of them! And nobody thinks twice about it. ◎ 2

You wouldn't tell people to just suck it up, to live with the pain and discomfort, or to just accept that it's a part of their lives. You would encourage them to seek help for something that is curable! So why should low mood be any different?

> ☻ Whatever the cause, if negative feelings don't go away, are too much for you to cope with, or are stopping you from carrying on with your normal life, you may need to make some changes and get some extra support. Making small changes in your life, such as resolving a difficult situation, talking about your problems, or getting more sleep, can usually improve your low mood.[1]

The bottom line is this: Low mood is not something we have to get used to or live with. Instead, it is something that we can combat, and defeat, with the right tools.

* * *

RECAP ✎

- Low mood is not a figment of your imagination or something you can just snap out of.

- Low mood is not depression. Depression needs a combination of therapy and medication to recover from. Low mood can be improved by taking positive action and resolving issues that may be causing it.

---

[1] https://www.nhs.uk/conditions/stress-anxiety-depression/low-mood-and-depression/

- When we've been 'down' for an extended period of time, we can forget how to focus on and choose the things that make us happy on a daily basis.

- All emotions are important but when they linger longer than they should they can be debilitating, exhausting, and block the normal happiness of life out.

- Mental health, despite its huge stigma, is not a personal failing. Millions of people suffer from mood disorders worldwide. You are not alone.

LINKED TO

1. Social Butterfly

2. Give Me the Drugs!

WHATS PUSHING YOUR BUTTONS?

♪♫♪ FIGHT SONG — RACHEL PLATTEN ♪♫♪

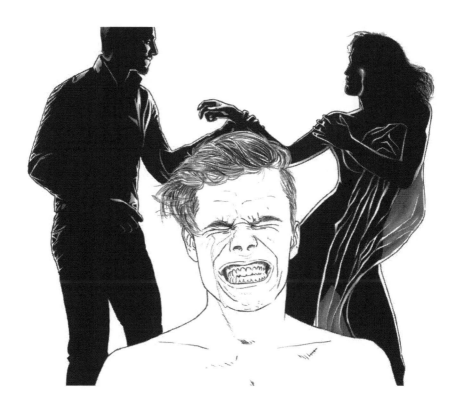

ARTWORK BY JAMES CRUMBO

Sometimes there is no known reason for your low mood. One day you just wake up and you're sad. Many different things can play a role, but the bottom line is, low mood can affect anyone. It doesn't matter who you are, where you live, how successful, loved, wealthy, or strong you are. Low mood doesn't differentiate.

Some people can pinpoint an exact incident that started them on a downward spiral, such as the death of a loved one. These are called 'triggers.' For others, triggers are hard to pinpoint. Sadness, anxiety, or anger just seem to creep up on them a little at a time.

Past experiences and present circumstances can both be triggers, and it's important to try and recognize yours. What makes you sad? Is there something in your past? Are you worried about your future? **Knowing what started or increases your sadness, and dealing with those issues, is vital to defeating low mood.**

There are so many things that can affect your emotions, and subsequently your mood. Some common triggers are:

- The stress of everyday life

- Loneliness

- Perfectionism

- Negative thinking

- Loss of a loved one

- Money issues

- Overwhelmed by world issues

- No sense of belonging

- Discontent

- Heritage

- Environment

- Physical abuse
- Emotional abuse
- Neglect
- Lack of pleasure in life
- Not connecting with other people
- Lack of love or touch
- Moving house
- Having children
- Lack of sleep or poor sleep habits
- Negative people in your life
- Not understanding yourself, or your personality type
- Changing jobs
- Energy loss
- Relationship breakup
- Ignoring your emotions
- The pressure to live up to people's expectations

The chapters in *Choosing Happy* will help you combat many of these triggers; however, some of them will need more specialized attention. If you've experienced abuse in your life, or you're going through things like relationship breakups, then you may want to seek professional help in addition to using this book.

A great way to address triggers is by using something called a cognitive loop or 'trigger loop.' ▶ Trigger loops look at what began your reaction - your trigger. They then look at the negative thought that causes the emotion we attach to that thought, and the behaviour we then exhibit. Trigger - Negative thought – Emotion - Behaviour.

Working through trigger loops after the fact helps us to see what we could have done differently, so that next time it happens, we can break the loop. Here's an example: You receive a message from your friend saying she can't make your planned catch-up. Sorry. You immediately think you must have done something wrong. This makes you sad and anxious. You begin to ruminate on every interaction you've shared with your friend recently to try and puzzle out why she doesn't want to catch up.

When you reflect on this loop you can find better ways to address it. You can't alter your friend's message, but you can change your reaction to it. Instead of immediately thinking the worst you can challenge your negative thoughts with fact and instead think of 3 'alternate truths' for why she may have cancelled. (We talk more about this in 'A Positive Spin on Negative Thoughts' 🔗1) You can use smiling🔗2 and affirmations🔗3 to boost your mood and try tapping🔗4 to break any lingering rumination.

The most dangerous untruths are truths slightly distorted.
-GEORG CHRISTOPH LICHTENBURG-

Next time something similar triggers a reaction, you already know ways in which you can combat it. Having tools to combat your triggers is incredibly important and empowering. And the more often you use them, the easier it becomes to break that loop before it gets started.

☻ When a negative thought pops up in our mind, it usually triggers an emotion, like sadness or anger, and it's only by questioning those thoughts that you can find out why you feel the way you do. By doing so, you delve deeper into what's stored in your subconscious (and why it's there). This is necessary, especially if you need to clear out some of those thoughts and let them go.[2]

Overcoming low mood means understanding your triggers and dealing with them, whether it's stress, negative thoughts, past experiences, or exhaustion. It means reclaiming the parts of yourselves you have ignored for years, and accepting that low mood is not a failing, but a problem you can combat. Then, and only then, can you begin to defeat your low mood, and appreciate what it means to be a whole, well, happy person.

* * *

RECAP ✄

- Low mood doesn't differentiate. It doesn't care where you live or how successful, loved, wealthy or strong you are. It affects everyone the same.

- Past experiences and present circumstances can all be triggers. Some common triggers are loneliness, perfectionism, negative thinking, loss of a loved one, money issues and lack of pleasure in life.

- If you've experienced abuse or you are going through a relationship breakup you may want to seek professional help in addition to using this book.

---

[2] https://www.consciouslifestylemag.com/negative-thoughts-getting-rid-of/

- Having tools to combat your triggers is incredibly important as overcoming low mood means understanding and dealing with your triggers.

- A great way to address triggers is by using a 'trigger loop'. They look at what began your emotion – your trigger. Then they look at the negative thoughts, the emotion, and the behaviour that follows. Trigger - Negative thought – Emotion - Behaviour. When you assess and reflect on these loops they can help you react differently to similar situations in the future.

ACTION STEPS ✎

Do now:

- Start by writing a trigger list of everything you can think of in your life that may be a trigger. Use the list above to prompt you, but remember it is in no way exhaustive. Keep your list somewhere accessible because you're going to be adding to it.

Plan to:

- Write a list of things you could do to help combat these triggers. You can add to this list as you work your way through *Choosing Happy* and work out what things work best for you. There is a printable graph you can use on my website www.how2without.com, as shown in the example below.

- Next, set an hourly alarm for daylight hours. Every hour when it chimes, stop what you're doing and assess your feelings. If you're feeling down, try to pinpoint what triggered it. Add this trigger to your 'trigger list.'

- After you've assessed your feelings I want you to work your way through a trigger loop and reflect on what happened, and how you could have reacted differently. Smile (especially if you don't feel like it) and repeat an affirmation in your head.

Work toward:

- Combating your triggers with the suggestions in this book, and if needed, professional help.

LINKED TO

1. A Positive Spin on Negative Thoughts

2. Smile – Your Face Won't Crack

3. Say it Like You Mean it

4. The Weird and the Wonderful

TRIGGER TABLE

Lack of sleep-exhaustion	Use a meditation app	Deal with emotional issues.	See GP about iron levels and thyroid	Try eating and drinking Tryptophan foods before bed	Reduce your caffeine intake
Negative thoughts	Pick and use affirmations	Understand rumination and how to beat it	Challenge your thoughts. Use facts	Practice meditation	Use tapping to break the rumination cycle
Loneliness	Join a group or club	Make socializing part of every week	Connect with like-minded people online	Stop to say hello to people at the shops	Spend quality time with people you love
Money issues	Write a budget	Get rid of unnecessary expenses	Understand your weekly spend	Use cash instead of credit cards	Consider alternative or extra work
Lack of love or touch	Instigate sex with your partner	Start every day by hugging your children	Make a point of touching your partner several times every day	Learn the art of self-pleasure	Be kind to yourself. Love yourself first
Stress	Practice meditation every day	Exercise every day	Make time for yourself	Learn how to fully relax	Learn to live in the moment

HAPPY HAPPY JOY JOY
♪♫♪ HAPPY — PHARREL WILLIAMS ♪♫♪

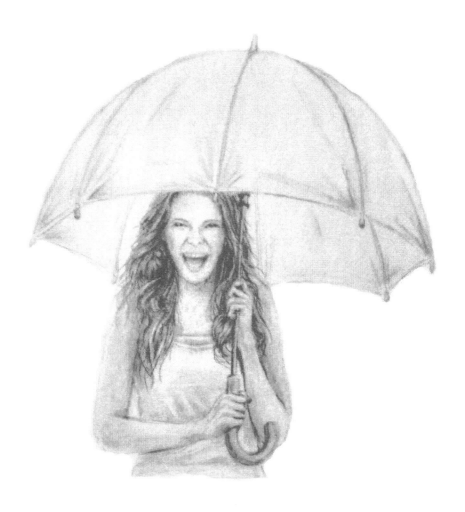

ARTWORK BY CRAIG DAWSON

Happiness. It's a rather unambiguous word. Everyone knows what it means, and we've all felt it at some point in our lives, but what is it really? What is it that makes us happy? And how do we hold on to happiness once we've found it?

You're not the only one who's confused about happiness. In fact, what happiness truly means is still highly debated. Probably because it's different for every person.

> *More than simply positive mood, happiness is a state of well-being that encompasses living a good life—that is, with a sense of meaning and deep satisfaction.* [3]

What we do know for certain is what it's not.

We know it's not material possessions or wealth. **Science has proven time and again that it is not 'things' that bring happiness.** In fact, some of the happiest people in the world are those that have the least.

Psychology professor Tim Kasser has been researching how materialism impacts our well-being for over 25 years and this is what he has to say, "Studies show that the more people prioritize materialistic values, the less happy they are. They are less satisfied with their lives, they feel less vital and energetic, and they are less likely to experience pleasant emotions like happiness, contentment, and joy."[4]

---

[3] https://www.psychologytoday.com/basics/happiness
[4] http://thepsychreport.com/conversations/materially-false-qa-tim-kasser-pursuit-good-goods/

It's not success that makes us happy either. We've been taught that when we *succeed* (in our jobs, goals, and relationships), we'll be happy. But the reality is, the opposite is true. The *happier* you are, the likelier you are to be successful, to have a loving marriage, be wealthy, even healthier than others. Happiness makes success more likely.

Happiness is also not entirely genetics. You've heard people say, 'That girl was born smiling.' That's actually true! Some people are just happier than others. Genetics account for a whopping 50% of how happy you are naturally (your set or starting point), but your set point can be altered.[5]▶ This is something that scientists are just starting to discover, but it means that if you're born with a naturally glum perspective, you *can* change it.

> ☻ "Happiness is genetically influenced but not genetically fixed. The brain's structure can be modified through practice. If you really want to be happier than your grandparents provided for in your genes, you have to learn the kinds of things you can do, day by day, to bounce your set point up and avoid the things that bounce it down." -UNIVERSITY OF MINNESOTA PROFESSOR EMERITUS OF PSYCHOLOGY DAVID LYKKEN, PHD-

According to a recent study[6], the more we focus on helping others, without any agenda of our own, the happier we seem to become in the long run (upping our set point). This could be because the more we begin to value others, the more value we give ourselves. Essentially, you're boosting your self-esteem by

---

[5] https://link.springer.com/article/10.1007%2Fs11205-009-9559-x
[6] https://www.psychologytoday.com/us/blog/happiness-in-world/201304/how-reset-your-happiness-set-point

being kind to others, and increasing your base level of happiness into the bargain. It's win-win!

Is it harder to be happy when the deck is genetically stacked against you? Or if you're struggling financially or mentally? I think it takes more conscious effort, but I believe it is just as hard for someone who seemingly has everything to understand and hold onto happiness as it is for someone who has much less.

We in the Western world have such a skewed belief on what true happiness is, and how we can find it, that I think it is often harder for us to attain. Many people think if they just get that raise, lose a couple of dress sizes, buy the perfect house, and have a partner and children, then life will be grand.

The reality is though, when you reach a goal, you automatically move the goal posts. It's how we have evolved as humans, by constantly striving to better ourselves. But this trait isn't always helpful, because while the drive to have more helps us push ourselves, having more does *not* make us happier. 🖉1

So, if it's not success, wealth, or genetics that make us happy, then what the heck does? And when was the last time you even stopped to think about that? Because if you did, you could probably pinpoint many things that make you happy quite accurately. And I doubt they'd be the big-ticket items society would have us believe.

You see, happiness can be created by experiencing pleasurable moments in your life. What those moments are, are different for every person. Because of this, part of learning to be happy is understanding yourself. You need to figure out what you really love in life, and what your body, mind, and soul need to not only function, but grow.

If you know which activities and experiences provide you with happiness, you are able to seek them out and participate in them whenever you like. This allows you to have moments of happiness frequently, and on demand, as it were. And it is these little things in life, much more than the big ones, that help you feel well, whole, and happy.

For some people, being around family and friends makes them happy. For others, patting their pet brings them happiness. For some it is shopping, music, exercise, or dancing. Find which activities work for you, and ensure you are participating in at least one of them every single day. Don't worry, we go through a stack of these in the following chapters.

Happiness is about more than just doing the things you love, though. It's about making the most of the good times, being grateful and content with what we have, and learning how to create happiness from every experience. There are so many things in our day-to-day lives that can bring us happiness. Be willing to try new things, take risks, and explore your world.

Because while it's great knowing which activities make you happy, it's been shown that the happiest people are actually those who get out of their own comfort zones. ▶ They do things that they're not sure about, or that terrify them a little, and they push the boundaries. They don't play it safe or stick to only those activities they *know* they'll enjoy. They try new experiences, learn new things, and grow as people. ✆ 2

And the people who are curious about life and put themselves out there are also the people who engage in other happiness activities more often. Things like practicing gratitude and smiling.

"Sometimes happiness is a feeling, sometimes it's a decision."

Learning to be happy means changing the way we perceive and react to everything in life and making happiness a conscious decision. You see, humans as a whole are preoccupied with happiness, and yet we don't make it a priority in our lives. It's not something we think about or make time for. If anything, we are mostly happy by accident. It's not a conscious decision on our end at all. But it should be!

Like many things in life, happiness needs to be continuously worked on. Just like you wouldn't enter a marathon without training, and expect to win, you can't expect to become happy overnight. You can't force it. But you can practice it. Every day. Because the more we prioritize happiness, the easier it becomes.

So, if all it takes to be happy is to choose to be, then why can't we all just stop what we're doing, decide to be happy, and live out the rest of our lives as merry as can be?

Well, you have to allow yourself to be happy, for a start.

It seems silly, doesn't it? If anyone had asked me 2 years ago if I wanted to be happy I would have said yes. Of course! I just didn't know how.

We had an horrendous year a while back where we went to 7 funerals, and subconsciously I think I thought that it wasn't okay to be happy when others were grieving. I felt like I needed to be sad. That if I was happy and smiling, it would somehow diminish that loss.

On top of that I was doing round after round of fertility treatments. And every single one of them failed. I blamed myself. I was angry, and bitter, and incredibly sad. I must have been doing something wrong. Perhaps I was exercising too much. Perhaps I wasn't exercising enough. Surely this was a sign that I was a terrible mother and I shouldn't actually have more children?

Everything I did in my day-to-day life seemed to be tainted with all these emotions. Even when I was with people I loved, and that loved me, I was sad. And in a warped kind of way I felt like if I wasn't, then it meant I didn't care. And so, I clung to my sadness, until I forgot how to be happy.

Now I can see where I went wrong. Happiness is not about laughing in the face of grief, or anger, or disappointment. It is about feeling those emotions, acknowledging them and dealing with them, but ultimately moving on from them. It's about choosing to focus on the good in your life instead of the bad.

Allowing myself to be happy meant that I had to learn to let go of the sadness, the hurt, and the guilt that I was carrying around with me. And I had a surprising amount for someone who from the outside was doing so well.

> *"The key to being happy is knowing you have the power to choose what to accept and what to let go."*
> -DODINSKY-

If you are carrying around guilt, sadness, disappointment, fear, anger, or pain, then you will constantly be weighed down and bombarded by these feelings. Because whatever baggage we're carrying around directly influences our happiness simply by being present.

Overcoming low mood means dealing with your stress, your negative thoughts, and your distorted way of seeing things. It means reclaiming the parts of ourselves we have ignored for years and giving ourselves permission to be happy. It means building up happiness pathways and prioritizing them! It means letting go of society's warped ideas of happiness and discovering what brings *us* joy.

Because being happy is the first step to experiencing true joy. Happiness provides us with a boost in energy, a love of life, people, and experiences, but eventually these moments fade. Happiness is unlike joy in the fact that you can find it for a moment, and in the next be sad again. Joy, on the other hand, exists even on bad days and in bad situations.

True joy▶ comes from really knowing yourself, from embracing who you are and being content with it, and from living an open, loving existence. True joy is long lasting, accessible even in tough times, and fed by your happiness. And that kind of joy is the ultimate goal. But happiness is a great start!

We all know how to be happy. It's an intrinsic part of us. It's just that many of us are out of practice. This is your opportunity to rediscover what makes *you* happy. Grab it! Because happiness is powerful, and life-changing. But it can only ever be sourced internally. You have to choose happiness for yourself.

* * *

RECAP 📌

- Happiness does not come from material possessions or wealth. It does not grow through success and it's not even entirely genetics (although these account for 50% of our happiness).

- It is just as hard for someone who seemingly has everything to be happy than for those who have much less.

- Happiness can be created by experiencing pleasurable moments in your life. Figure out what you really love, no matter how small and do them! This could be patting a pet, being around family and friends, shopping, music, or exercise.

- Happiness is about making the most of the good times, being grateful and content with what we have, and learning how to create happiness from every experience.

- Happiness needs to be continually worked on. Prioritize it and practice it every day.

- Being happy is powerful and life-changing and the first step to experiencing true joy. But it can only ever be sourced internally. You have to allow yourself to be happy.

ACTION STEPS ✏️

Do now:

- Happiness is experienced differently by every person, and different things make each of us happy. Consider doing an online test to see if you are an introvert or an extrovert. Many things an extrovert will find exhilarating will make an introvert exhausted. Finding out what works for you as an individual is incredibly important.

- Write a list of all the things in your life that make you happy. Even the little things. Heck, especially the little things! Because it's the little things that happen often enough to really influence us on a daily basis.

Your happy things can be as simple as:

- A sunny day

- Someone smiling at you

- Patting a pet

- Seeing a blooming flower

- Smelling fresh coffee

- Completing a task

- Hearing your favourite song

You could also add bigger things like:

- Visiting a friend

- Swimming at the beach

- Creating or crafting something new

- Mountain Biking

- Going out to dinner

- Watching a favourite movie

- Having an entire day to yourself (sign me up!)

Plan to:

- Work at least one thing that makes you happy into your daily routine. This will help you discover joy daily and build happiness pathways.

- Branch out! Try something new, exciting, or even a bit terrifying, even if you're not sure you'll like it. Be curious.

Work towards:

- Being happy many times a day, every day. This is both easier and harder than it seems, but you *will* get there.

LINKED TO

1. Aim for the Stars

2. Learning to Grow

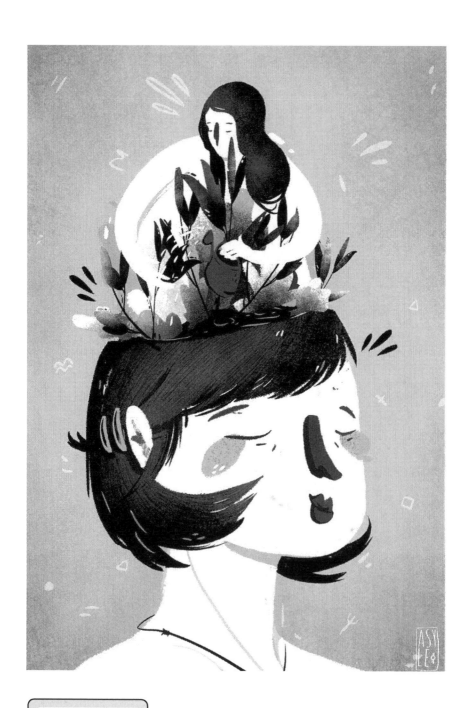

ARTWORK BY ASYLE

MIND

OUR MIND IS AN INCREDIBLE TOOL. BUT IT IS NOT INFALLIBLE. LIKE A COMPUTER IT CAN BE PROGRAMMED, BUT THIS MEANS IT RELIES ON YOU TO INPUT THE INFORMATION IT NEEDS. AND UNFORTUNATELY, PAST AND PRESENT EXPERIENCES, NEGATIVE THOUGHTS AND BELIEFS CAN ALL DISTORT THE INFORMATION WE FEED OUR BRAIN.

RE—PROGRAMMING OUR MINDS WITH POSITIVE THOUGHTS IS A BIG PART OF OVERCOMING LOW MOOD. IT'S NOT EASY OVERWRITING THINGS WE'VE THOUGHT AND HOW WE'VE SPOKEN FOR YEARS, BUT IT IS ACHIEVABLE!

EMOTIONAL ROLLERCOASTER
♪♫♪ WALKING ON SUNSHINE — KATRINA AND THE WAVES ♪♫♪

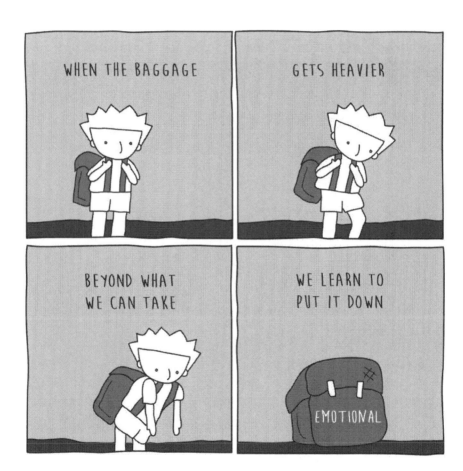

ARTWORK BY MJ.OANNE

> *Our emotions need to be as educated as our intellect. It is important to know how to feel, how to respond, and how to let life in so that it can touch you.*
> - JIM ROHN -

Emotions can be complicated, messy, and debilitating. But they can also be helpful, cathartic, and incredible. To survive the emotional rollercoaster that our lives can become you need to remember a few things though.

- We need all our emotions, even the rough ones ✆ 1

- Emotions were never meant to be long-lived

- Other people's problems can only be addressed by themselves

- You *can* overcome lingering or negative emotions

Let's take a closer look at some of the main stumbling blocks people face.

Whose problem is it?

I have a serious problem separating other people's issues from my own. Even when it was something that was obviously not my problem, I would try to fix it. Which is not necessarily a bad thing. We should all help others where we can. Except, I was focusing on others to the exclusion of my own happiness. And often over things that I couldn't change. Many things in other people's lives can only be dealt with by themselves (funnily enough).

People's attitudes, the way they interacted with me, the choices they made, and situations that occurred around me, I stressed about them all. Why had they made that atrocious decision (again)? Why were they so hateful? What could I do to help them? Round and round those thoughts would go. But there were never any clear answers. Why? Because they weren't my problems to solve.

My husband has a catch phrase I want to share with you. It changed how I reacted to situations and gave me clarity. It's simple, as all good things are, but oh, so powerful.

"Whose problem is it?"

It can be applied to any situation. Is a work colleague being nasty? *Whose problem is it?* Is a family member being childish? *Whose problem is it?* Is a friend being petty? *Whose problem is it?* Often, we personalize 2 everything that happens in our lives, when in reality, it's nothing to do with us at all.

Yes, people might be directing their anger, nastiness, or apathy our way, but it's not caused by us (unless you're being an A-hole, in which case, pull your head in!). And because it's not our emotion, it can't be fixed by us. Instead it's something that they need to deal with themselves.

It is up to others to create lasting change in their own lives, and while you can help them, they need to be the driving force behind it. Imagine you are trying to push a massive boulder across a field. You might make it a short distance, but the struggle will leave you feeling drained. Now imagine the boulder has wheels and an engine. It is doing most of the work itself, you're just guiding it around the pot holes.

Asking yourself, *'Whose problem is it?'* allows us to separate other people's issues from our own lives, distance ourselves, and not get sucked into a vortex of emotions that we can't control - because they were nothing to do with us in the first place. Instead you can learn to see them as issues that have been forced on you by association, guilt, or familial ties. Sometimes all three!

Help where you can, but make sure the ball is firmly in their court. It is *not* your problem. And while that seems selfish, learning to separate yourself from other people's issues is an important part of finding personal happiness. Everyone makes their own choices in life. Don't let other people's anger, bitterness, or hate influence how you feel about yourself, or live your life.

Guilt

Guilt is debilitating, and yet we are all 'guilty' (pun intended) of carrying it around with us. Some guilt serves a purpose. It allows us to see where things are wrong and address them, but most guilt is just worthless baggage. It's like taking a bikini to Antarctica. You won't need it, but you have trouble leaving it behind.

Not only does guilt hold us back from enjoying life, it can warp the way we actually view life, and the interactions we have with others.

Like I said, guilt is debilitating.

But how do we escape it? It seems like there's always something to feel guilty about. The ice-cream after dinner, not making time for friends, a stray thought, not reaching a goal, or simply not being enough. The answer is that you don't. You will always feel guilt at one time or another. It's how you address it that's key.

First, stop ignoring your guilt. Instead, have a good look at it. If it helps, write down everything you're feeling guilty about. Now, focus on just one of those areas of guilt. Ask yourself:

- Did you actually do anything wrong?

- Can you do anything to remedy the situation?

- Is your guilt based on your own life standards, or someone else's?

Sometimes feelings of guilt take hold simply because we contemplated doing something, or a thought popped into our heads which we quickly dismissed. Even though we didn't act on our thoughts, we feel guilty for them! Let this guilt go. Everyone thinks about doing things they shouldn't, it's human nature to evaluate all our options, even subconsciously. But if you didn't follow through with it, then forgive yourself. You're not the villain you've made yourself out to be.

Feeling guilt on a much stronger level than necessary is called neurotic guilt. It's classified by feeling guilty about things you cannot change, and can arise from self-doubt, or childhood events, or by not doing something when others think you should. You need to clarify whether your guilt is valid or not, and based on this, either work at fixing the problem causing you guilt, or learn to let it go.

If you feel guilty about the same things on a regular basis, then you may need to address why. Is this because you're actually doing something wrong and it's conflicting with your moral compass? Or are you contemplating something you know is wrong? Sometimes our guilt does exactly what it needs to do and stops us making mistakes we can't undo. It's another way our conscience prompts us to do the right thing.

These questions can help you decide if your guilt is founded or not, and what actions you're going to take:

- Who would your actions benefit or harm?

- Would this thing bring you lasting, or fleeting happiness?

- Is your guilt based on personal standards, or other people's?

- Would the action be worth the consequences?

Sometimes we get so caught up in feelings of guilt that we can't see clearly. If you're having trouble figuring out whether your guilt is founded or not, think about speaking with a trusted friend or family member, and getting their opinion on the situation.

Do you actually have any reason to be feeling guilty, or do you just need to let it go? Listen to them!! We know our brains are not to be trusted sometimes. Feeling guilty for no reason is not going to help the situation, but it can do you a lot of harm. Let it go.

If you have done something to feel guilty about, then stop sweeping it under the carpet! You're feeling guilty because you need to do something about it. If you can, right your wrong. Apologize for bad behaviour, make up for your actions in any way you can, accept responsibility if something is truly your fault, and then, most importantly, forgive yourself.

None of us are perfect. Goodness knows I've done things I've felt guilty about. But those things don't define me, any more than they define you. They are just moments in our lives. One amongst the many. Learn from your mistakes but don't let them colour your future.

> (★) Previously emotions have been considered relatively unchanging, basic, feeling states. Amodio's research presents a new idea of emotions serving a dynamic motivational function for regulating behaviour. [For example] although it feels bad, guilt plays a critical role in promoting prosocial behaviour. That worried feeling in our gut often serves as the impetus for our stab at redemption. [7]

Many of our 'guilts' are based on other people's beliefs, or on our upbringing, rather than things we actually believe ourselves. Catholic guilt is a perfect example, and a term most people know. It is used to show that a person's guilt is caused from set beliefs held by the Catholic church. And yet many people who feel Catholic guilt no longer align themselves with those beliefs. They are just so deeply entrenched in their psyche, they feel guilt regardless.

This kind of guilt does us a lot of harm, because we are constantly struggling with how we *want* our life to be vs how we *think* our life should be. Make sure your opinions are your own, not other people's. Work out your own set of values, and what's important to you, and let go of other people's grip on your life.

Carrying around unfounded guilt can stop you from enjoying life. It can overshadow friendships and relationships, it can make you think less of yourself - often for no reason at all - and cause you to choose paths you actually don't want your life to follow.

Guilt is a lot like the monsters under your bed. When you pretend they're not there they continue to bother you, to haunt your brain, and interfere with your life. When you face them

---

[7] https://www.sciencedaily.com/releases/2007/07/070724113727.htm

full on, you realise that they are not worth worrying about, and that you are blowing them completely out of proportion.

Focus light on your guilt, and it will stop lurking and come into focus. Ask yourself the questions above, do what needs to be done, and then let it go.

Worry

Are you a worry wort? Do you worry about things you've said and done? Do you worry about things that haven't happened yet and even things that have a high probability of NOT happening? This is me. Well, it was me. I'm pretty good now. I still worry, but I have ways of analysing and dealing with that worry, and that's what I want to talk about now.

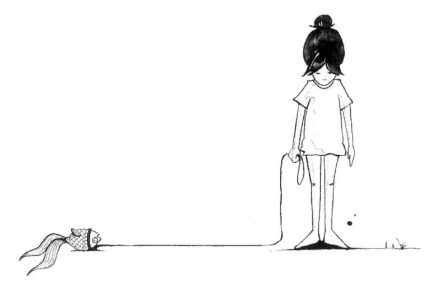

Worry, like guilt, can serve a purpose. Worrying about where your next pay check is coming from, or if your child is going to get sunburnt, or how you will do in your exams, these are all logical.

ARTWORK BY CAROLINE RUSS

They remind you of things that are happening in your life that (wait for it) *you can alter*. Worry was never meant to be an action-less feeling. It was meant to be a prompt. A reminder that something is happening that you need to take action on.

Do you need to job hunt, put sunscreen on your child, or study for exams? Then do it!

Worry should be a three-step process.

1. **Identify the worry**

2. **Solve the worry through action**

3. **Release the worry**

See what I did there in number three? Yup, not subtle at all. But just in case you missed it, I'm going to say it again. Release the worry. Holding onto worries once they're in the past is pointless. It just makes you stressed and unhappy. You've got to let it go.

If your child got sunburnt, then that sucks, but you can't do anything about it now. You just make a mental note to put on more sunscreen next time. Did you bomb out in your exams? Truly stink. But it's done. You need to let that worry go and look forward.

Think of solutions instead. Can you re-sit your exam? Does the grade on this exam matter for your career long-term? Can you build yourself up in a different area to compensate? These are all possible solutions to the problem, and this is where your thoughts would be better spent. Coming up with solutions and letting the worry fall by the wayside.

Worrying about money is the worst, especially when you can't see any solutions to the problem. And you know what?

Sometimes there aren't any for the immediate future. Sometimes you just have to keep on keeping on. And that can be an awful feeling. However, worrying does nothing to change this fact.

So instead of worrying, try making plans and setting goals ◎ 3. What can you do now to ensure you have a better future financially? You can't budget your way out of being broke. But you also can't worry your way out of it.

Worry can highlight a problem, but it can't fix it. That takes action.

So again:

1. Identify the worry

2. Solve the worry through action

3. Release the worry

While this doesn't solve the fact that you're broke, it does give you a clear head for figuring out what to do. Remember that no change is instantaneous, so be patient, review your goal and alter when necessary, and make small changes and time investments every day. You will get there!

RECAP ✄

- You cannot control other people's emotions. Asking yourself *"Whose problem is it?"* allows us to separate their issues from our own lives instead of taking them all on board.

- Some guilt serves a purpose, but most is just worthless baggage. It's how you address it that's key. Focus on what you feel guilty about. Did you actually do anything wrong? Can you do anything to remedy the situation? Is your guilt based on your own life standards or someone else's? Take action, let it go, and most importantly, forgive yourself.

- Worry, like guilt, can serve a purpose, but it was never meant to be an action-less feeling. Worry should be a 3-step process.

1. Identify the worry.

2. Solve the worry through action.

3. Release the worry.

ACTION STEPS ✎

Do now:

- Think of one worry you have. Identify what it is, and why you have it. Solve the problem through action and release the worry. Use affirmations ⊘4 and tapping ⊘5, etc., to stop your brain circling back to this problem. If your brain does circle back, think about the action you took to solve the problem so that your brain has a chance to recognize it no longer needs to worry about this issue.

Plan to:

- Apply the 'whose problem is it' mantra to any negative thoughts that occur after interactions with other people and their lives.

- Address your guilt by writing down anything you feel guilty about. Look at each item on your list and assess why you feel guilty, if it is founded, and what actions you can take to resolve it.

- When you find yourself worrying apply the 3-step process.

1. Identify the worry

2. Solve the worry through action

3. Release the worry

Work towards:

- Using the 'whose problem is it' mantra while in difficult situations.

- Using guilt as a valuable tool to keep you on the right path rather than a rod to beat yourself with.

- Identifying, solving and releasing worries as they occur.

LINKED TO

1. Lessons in Low Mood

2. A Positive Spin on Negative Thoughts

3. Aim for the Stars

4. Say It Like You Mean It

5. The Weird and the Wonderful

THINKING TOO MUCH ABOUT CRAP YOU SHOULDN'T

♪♫♪ I'M STILL STANDING — TARON EGERTON ♪♫♪

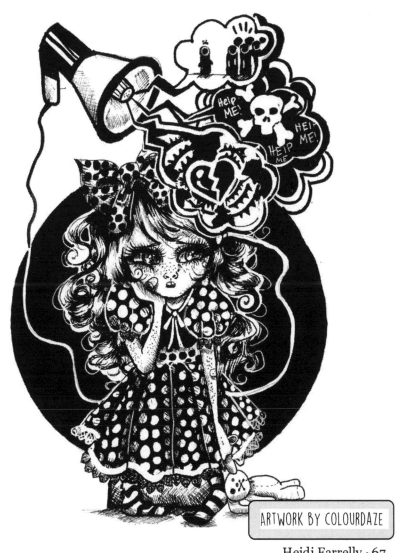

ARTWORK BY COLOURDAZE

If you read only one chapter in *Choosing Happy*, make sure it's this one. Because if someone had told me about rumination and how to overcome it several years ago, life would have been a lot simpler.

When I first found out I had depression I did a lot of research on other people's journey with it. And one of the little books I read really stuck with me. It was called *Love Yourself - Like Your Life Depends on It*, by Kamal Ravikant▶. It was neither expensive nor widely acclaimed (although it did have a large number of positive reviews), and it spoke of the author's battle, and ultimate victory, over depression. Look it up - it's well worth a read.

One of the main things Kamal talked about was rumination. Never heard of it? Neither had I. Do you have a negative thought, and then think about it constantly, or find it running through your mind without consciously bringing it up? This is rumination. And I am so good at it. And the more I talk to people who suffer from low mood, sadness, and depression, the more I realise it's something many of us are very good at!

However, while we might be awesome at it, it's not doing us any favours. In fact, I would go so far as to say it is the number one thing that dragged me deeper into sadness and depression than I had ever been before.

You see, rumination (or thinking way too much about crap that we shouldn't care about), takes a perfectly normal thought, and focuses all your attention on it. It then pushes, and pokes, and pulls at it, in an attempt to 'better understand it,' when in actual fact it just helps you hold onto all your negative thoughts and revisit them, over, and over, again.

The tricky thing about rumination is that it feels like it's helpful, but there's no action taken, and you don't move forward to some sort of solution.
-CARLA GRAYSON-

And when we are sad, low, or depressed, the thoughts on loop in our minds are usually not happy ones. It might be simple things like, 'I am not good at anything,' or 'My life is crap.' Perhaps it's 'I'm ugly,' or 'I hate myself.' Maybe it's something someone said to you, or you thought was implied. The bottom line is this, though: The more you think about (ruminate) on these things, the more power you give them.

Kamal describes rumination as pathways. The more you walk a particular path, the more defined it becomes, the easier it is to walk, and the more likely we are to return to it. When you go to bed, when you're driving to work, when you're doing dishes, when you're out with friends, your thoughts are on a perpetual loop in your head. And every time that loop repeats, it engraves itself more deeply in your mind.

Your brain is smart. And it's capable of creating new pathways based on the information you provide it with. But like a computer, it is only as good as the information you download to it.

Think of your brain like Wikipedia. It receives information from its author - you. Your Wiki brain then tells you (the visiting person) that all this information is true, because that's what it was provided with.

And **even when you know that information is distorted or incorrect, the more you ruminate on a subject, the**

more 'true' your brain believes it is. So, then it provides 'hyperlinks' (defined pathways) to that Wiki page so you can access it more quickly, because you seem to be visiting it a lot. The more you read that page, the truer it starts to feel, until you can no longer differentiate between fact and fiction.

> ☢ Self-reflection can have both light and dark sides. Nonetheless, there is a form of self-reflection that has harmful consequences and can lead to the magnification and prolongation of depressive moods. Ruminative response style is a form of responding to distress, which "involves repetitively and passively focusing on symptoms of distress and on the possible causes and consequences of these symptoms." [8]

Rumination is a bastard. It tricks you. It keeps you going over and over painful things. Things that are better off forgotten and moved on from. It aids you in building conversations and arguments in your mind about things that haven't even happened yet! It encourages you to believe the worst about yourself and others, all while cementing these thoughts into your head as facts to be believed at all costs.

But just as you can edit Wikipedia with new information, so too can you edit your brain.

Until I studied rumination, I used to have real trouble switching off those negative thoughts that were looping around my brain. I'm sure you know it's almost impossible to just 'stop thinking.' The trick is to overwrite those negative thoughts instead, with a mantra or affirmation, instead of trying to switch off altogether. The idea is to make the loop path of your

---

[8] https://www.ncbi.nlm.nih.gov/pmc/articles/PMC5153413/

mantra deeper than the other paths, so it becomes the new 'go to' for your brain. Kamal used the affirmation 'I love myself.'

Whenever he started to ruminate, Kamal would start repeating 'I love myself,' 'I love myself,' over and over in his head. A mantra helps by taking over from those negative thoughts and helping your brain to focus on something positive. In his case, 'I love myself.'

It doesn't matter if you don't entirely believe what you're saying at first. The only thing that matters is challenging, and breaking, that train of thought. The more you repeat your mantra, the more engraved this new positive pathway will become in your brain, until this is what you will think subconsciously. Remember, your brain believes the information it is provided with, so provide it with something positive!

You might want to start with a milder affirmation such as 'I like myself.' For some people, going from profoundly negative thoughts to such positive ones is too big a jump. Check out Affirmations 1 for more details. But the premise is the same. Essentially, fake it 'til you make it!

This was a game changer for me! I have always thought about things far more than I should and read far more into people's comments than I needed to. I would have fictitious arguments with people in my head, on the off chance they would happen, because I hated not knowing what to say. And I revisited all the nasty comments, bad reviews, and any conversations I felt were 'lacking' to try and make sense out of them or see where I went wrong.

The reality is there will always be things that didn't pan out how you planned. Nasty things that were said in anger, or conversations and situations that just didn't make sense. But revisiting them will not change that! All it does is cement them in your mind and make you miserable. The trick is to combat them instead.

Some people may find they don't need a mantra, that just developing an awareness of rumination is enough. And in fact, this is a major battle in itself! Once you know you are doing something it is much easier to combat it. You can shake yourself out, give yourself a talking to, distract yourself with something else, whatever works.

My point is, knowing that rumination can be a dangerous and slippery slope, and identifying it early, can be as effective for some as an affirmation.

But for those who find awareness is simply not enough (like me), choose a mantra. It doesn't have to be 'I love myself.' This was important to Kamal because he hated himself and questioned whether he should be in the world. I chose 'I am AWESOME!' because I didn't value myself and my achievements. This was important to me. Find something that calls to you.

Then, start repeating your mantra to yourself when you wake up, or when you're brushing your teeth. Set an hourly alarm and when it sounds, take whatever you're thinking and replace it with your mantra. When you start having negative thoughts - say your mantra. When you're having fictitious conversations - say your mantra. Until you hear your alarm go off one day and realise the only thing you're thinking - is your mantra.

If the one thing you take away from this book is how to stop rumination in its tracks, then I will be supremely happy. **Remember, the more you think about something, the more it becomes a part of you.** What do you want written on your heart?

* * *

RECAP 📌

- Rumination (thinking too much) takes a perfectly normal thought and focuses all your attention on it. It helps you to hold onto all your negative thoughts and revisit them over and over again.

- It's almost impossible to just stop thinking negative thoughts so instead you need to learn to overwrite them. Your brain is smart and it's capable of creating new thought pathways based on the information you provide it with.

- Affirmations are a great way to overwrite your negative thoughts. You don't have to believe what you're saying at first, because the more you tell yourself something, the truer your brain will believe it is. Essentially, fake it 'til you make it!

ACTION STEPS ✎

Do now:

- Choose a mantra/affirmation that is important to you. Make sure it is short and easy to say, such as: I am loved, I am needed, I will be okay, this will pass.

Plan to:

- Set an hourly alarm and every time it rings replace whatever you're thinking about with your mantra. If hourly alarms aren't going to work, then incorporate your mantra into your daily routine. Say it when you're in the shower, when you first wake up, or when you go to bed.

Work towards:

- Using your mantra consciously to combat anger, stressful situations, sadness and anxiety.

- Using your mantra subconsciously in place of negative, or 'busy' thoughts.

LINKED TO

1. Say it Like you Mean It

JUST STOP IT

♪♫♪ TUBTHUMPING (I GET KNOCKED DOWN) — CHUMBAWAMBA ♪♫♪

Don't let your past dictate who you are but let it be a lesson that strengthens the person you'll become.

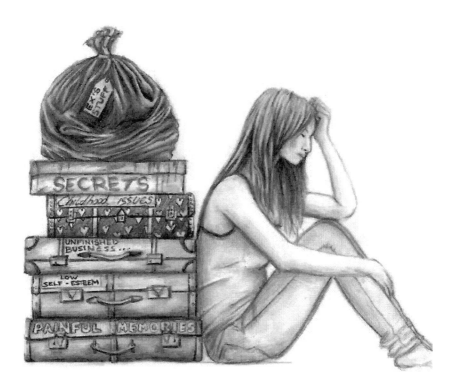

ARTWORK BY CRAIG DAWSON

My sister-in-law is fabulous with people. She is an excellent listener, but she's also not afraid to tell it like it is. As such, she does a lot of marriage and relationship mentoring, and she is really good at it. But sometimes when people are wallowing in their misery, when they are dredging up their past and existing on it like it's some exotic food group they just can't get enough of, she gets pissed.

She told me that sometimes she just wants to reach out and shake them, and say, "Just stop it!"

And this is exactly what I want to say to you. Stop it! Stop blaming your present on your past. Stop wallowing in your sadness and despair. Stop playing the victim of your own life. Stop giving your past and the people who have hurt you so much power!

Just stop it!

The more you allow yourself to re-live the bad times, to focus only on the things that aren't working in your life, the more likely you are to end up living with depression instead of just low mood. And believe me when I say it is just not worth it.

Humans by nature are selfish people. We have an instinctual urge to put ourselves first, to protect ourselves, and to survive. Our brains are literally wired for it! So, I get it. You're important. And your past experiences are also important. But they are not who you are. Yes, the past shapes and to some extent defines who we are today, but we can choose in what WAY it shapes us, for better or for worse.

Don't get me wrong, I know the things in our past have a way of overwhelming us and forcing themselves in our faces. We've talked about how they can be triggers for low mood, and the reason we are suffering in the first place. But past emotions can act like poison. You can't just push them down or ignore them, or they'll spread and fester.

Our past is something we need to face, and to deal with, instead of letting it rule and define our lives. **You can have a crap past and still rise above it.** It takes effort, and perseverance, and it's not easy. But it can be done. You just have to take it one step at a time. Because the truth is, we can never truly be happy while we're still holding on to our past. You have the ability to change. To rise above. To exceed all expectations – even your own. You are amazing.

So just stop it!

Move on. Leave the past where it belongs – in the past. Learn from your experiences, but don't cling to them. Grieve, but don't become your grief. Let go of your anger, your hate, and your bitterness. They no longer serve a purpose. The only thing these emotions are doing now is holding you back, and just like sadness they are supposed to be short-lived. They help us see and respond to dangerous or unhealthy situations. But they are not meant to be a part of our lives long-term.

So just stop it!

We become what we focus on. When we focus on happy things we become happy, when we focus on sad things we become sad, and when we focus on the past we become the sum of the emotions we find there. Angry, bitter, and disappointed. It truly is that simple.

When I was battling low mood, focusing on the negative events in my life not only helped me hold onto them, it made me more and more unable to move forward with and enjoy my life. But I got so used to only seeing the bad, and living with sadness as a daily companion, it just became comfortable! Not in a good way, but in the way you get used to a persistent headache. It's not pleasant, but you just accept it's there to stay.

My mood wasn't dictated by what was going wrong in my life, the things people had done to hurt me, and my past experiences. Yes, those things can have a negative effect, of course they can! But they don't control you unless you let them. My low mood was of my own making.

Unknowingly, unintentionally, I was perpetuating the cycle of my own low mood. And it was up to me to fix it. We are not destined to live out the life we have lived previously. Our lives are our own, and while some people have more choices than others, and some have an easier route, every single person has choice. You can choose which parts of your past you will allow into your present, and into your future.

So just stop it!

I know that's easier said than done. I understand you may have lived a horrible life, and you feel like you have no choices, and no strength. I mean, let's face it, your brain hamstrung you from the beginning. It created core circuits and pathways▶ from a young age to help you remember what you did wrong. Not because it hates you, but to remind you what NOT to do, to ensure your survival. ☍1

That's why it can be so hard to change the way we view and react to situations. Because that little gremlin in your brain is constantly pushing the refresh button! The good news is, your crappy past can make you stronger. Apparently, going through the wringer really *does* help you. Because it builds resilience.▶ You know, that ability to bounce back in tough times.

Focusing on past experiences and sources of personal strength can help you learn about what strategies for building resilience might work for you.[9]

And resilience is essential to finding happiness. Why? Because it gives us new perspective. Resilience teaches you to focus on what worked in stressful situations and what didn't, and use this knowledge to combat any stress, loss, or trauma you may encounter in your future. How bad-ass is that? Your past *can* have a profound impact on the person you become, but in a good way.

Bad situations will always happen. It's how we react to them, and learn from them, that makes all the difference.

So just stop it and move on with your life.

Yes, you might be hurting physically or mentally. Yes, your life might not be going to plan, but you are alive, you have the day at your feet, and only you control your thoughts and actions. How awesome is that? Stop complaining, criticizing, and gossiping, and instead find things to talk about that uplift you and those around you.

You have the power to create positive change, not just in yourself, but in all the lives that you touch.

So, what can you do if your life really is a series of unfortunate events? If there are no silver linings, or happy endings? You need to harden the heck up and stop feeling sorry for yourself,

9 http://www.apa.org/helpcenter/road-resilience.aspx

for a start. Seriously. Go read the gratitude section ⌾2 and then come back and tell me again that you have nothing in your life to be thankful for.

There are countless inspiring stories of people overcoming monumental events in their past and going on to achieve the impossible. Take Nick Vujicic,▶ for example. Nick was born with no arms and no legs. Here is a man who has every reason to be miserable and unhappy with his lot in life. And yet he is a world-renowned expert in living a joy-filled life despite your circumstances. He speaks with school groups as a motivational speaker, has written numerous books, and founded 2 companies.

But it's harder for young people, right? Wrong! Go and follow @lisacox.co on Instagram and prepare to be inspired. Lisa▶ is also a motivational speaker, a writer, and an author. Her feed is full of positivity and encouragement. And yet Lisa has been through more in her 27 years than you would believe. A brain haemorrhage, and subsequent pneumonia, heart attacks, and seizures left her dead. Twice!

Thankfully for us the doctors didn't give up on her, although she had to have 1 leg and all her toes amputated along with 9 fingertips. (She's super excited she got to keep the tenth!) All this damage to her brain left her with epilepsy, fatigue, and osteoarthritis and she is also 25% blind. And yet she is still a healthy, vibrant person that is actively encouraging and inspiring others with her positivity. She has definitely inspired me!

How do people like Nick and Lisa do it? They started by choosing to. That's all there is to it. And I know I'm going to get hate mail for this chapter, because there are people who simply will not agree with me. But unless you realize right now that you, and you alone, hold the power to change your life, no amount of hacks are going to help you.

Situations and events do impact our lives - of course they do. But they shouldn't define them or taint our present or our future. Instead, we need to learn how to address bad situations and see them for what they really are - one of the many occurrences in our lives. Just one.

And yes, that one thing may be horrific, and it may be followed by another one, but it still isn't the only thing that will ever happen in our lives. It's not the end of your story, just a part of it. And the problem with focusing on something, on giving it more attention than it deserves, is that it becomes a living, breathing 'thing' that sticks around far longer than it should.

> ☻ When difficult events occur, we can feel sorry for ourselves. This isn't helpful and will often drive us farther from where we want to be. Taking responsibility for your circumstances and not looking for ways to apportion blame enables you to seek out solutions. It is by far the most progressive and productive way to approach any adversity. Often you are more in control than you think; if you find yourself in the passenger seat, move into the driving seat and navigate your own way through whatever you are experiencing.[10]

What do parents always say about raising children (or animals!)? Don't reward bad behaviour with attention. And yet we are doing just that with bad situations. The more attention we give them, the more you 'feed' them, the more they grow.

---

[10] https://www.trainingjournal.com/articles/feature/resilience-—-essential-ingredient-happiness

Soon all you can see or think about is that one bad situation, and it blocks out any chance of sunshine entering your life.

You can choose how you view and react to every situation you find yourself in. You can choose right now that you will not be a reflection of your past, but that your past will be a stepping stone or a learning curve for a completely different future! You can choose who you socialize ✎ 3 with. You can choose to be grateful for the things you *do* have in your life. You can choose to wake up and greet a new day full of possibilities and promise. You can choose to agitate for change. You can choose to reach out for help. And you can choose to start dealing with your past, so you can get on with living your present. **You can choose to be happy.**

So just stop it!

You are an incredible person. You are strong enough to walk a new path. You are brave enough to face your demons and slay them. You have enough time to be grateful for what you have in life. You have enough money to keep your body alive and your brain functioning. You have enough health to be reading this book. People have done a lot more, with a lot less. Why should you be any different?

So just stop it!

Don't be the sum of your past. Live up to the possibilities of your future. And start moving towards an unfakably happy life.

* * *

RECAP ✎

- Past experiences are important. But they are not who you are. Our past is something we need to face and deal with, instead of letting it define our present and our future. Stop blaming your present on your past and giving people and events that have hurt you so much power!

- You are not destined to live out the life you have lived previously. Instead, you can choose which parts of your past you will allow into your present. You can choose to use your past experiences as learning curves, to rise above them, and exceed all expectations. Even your own. You are amazing.

- Emotions like grief, anger, hate and bitterness are not meant to be part of our lives long-term. The only thing these emotions are doing now is holding you back, and moulding you into an angry, bitter, sad person. Why? We become what we focus on.

- Resilience is the ability to bounce back in tough times. And resilience is essential to finding happiness because it teaches you to focus on what worked in stressful situations and what didn't. You can then use this knowledge to combat any stress, loss or trauma you may encounter in your future.

ACTION STEPS ✎

Do now:

- Think of times that were difficult in the past. Write them down, and then write down what helped you get through them. The situation, and the solution.

- Write your solutions into an easy-to-read list that you can break out and review whenever you're struggling with negative thoughts and emotions. Often the things that helped previously will help again.

- Smile! ⊘ 4 Believe me, for such a little thing it packs a big punch!

Plan to:

- Every time you catch yourself thinking about something from your past, think about one good or happy thing that has happened recently. It may be as simple as 'the sun came out today.' You may have noticed a tree in blossom, children having a snow fight (I hope you joined in!). Your favourite show might be one. You may have completed a chore you'd been putting off for ages. You may have exchanged smiles with a stranger or caught up with a friend.

- Whatever it is, focus on it. Think about what happened, how it made you feel. Smile, re-live it, and feel the happiness and joy, just like you did then. If you really can't think of a single positive thing that day, then think of something positive from your past. When you're done, remind yourself that life holds more than sadness for you. It is full of little joys, and happinesses (totally a word). You just need to find and focus on them. ⊘ 5

- When something is troubling you, address it. Have you been in this situation before? Look at the strategies you wrote down and see how you dealt with it last time.

- Shift your mood with a smile or laugh and look at the problem again from a different viewpoint. Often this new perspective will help you see and address your problem more easily.

- Tell yourself 3 alternate truths ⊘ 6 to help break the cycle of negativity.

- Work your way through *Choosing Happy* and add everything from it to your solutions list that you believe you could use when tackling difficult emotions from the past. Use this list to help you overcome old habits of holding onto past anger, sadness, and low mood.

- Make a list of goals 🔗 7 you would like to achieve in the future to encourage you to look forward.

- Plan things for your week that you know will make you happy, such as walking in nature, having coffee with a friend, or going for a swim.

Work towards:

- Dealing with, and letting go of, the pain, sadness, and anger of the past.

- Seeing the amazing things that are happening in your life right now.

- Anticipating the good things that are going to happen in your future.

LINKED TO 🔗

1. Thinking Too Much About Crap You Shouldn't

2. Great Attitude

3. Social Butterfly

4. Smile - Your Face Won't Crack

5. Mind Your Mind

6. A Positive Spin on Negative Thoughts

7. Aim for the Stars

A POSITIVE SPIN ON NEGATIVE THOUGHTS

♪♫♪ BISCUITS — KACEY MUSGRAVES ♪♫♪

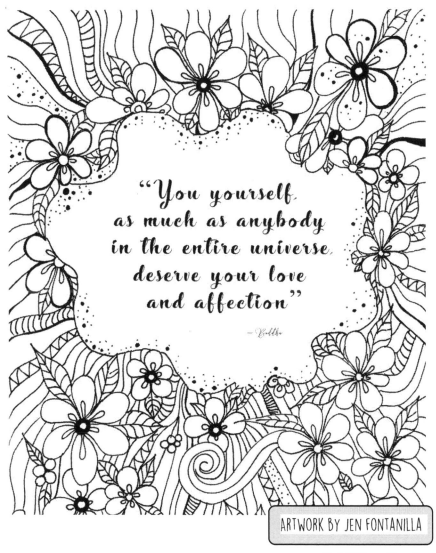

"You yourself,
as much as anybody
in the entire universe,
deserve your love
and affection"

— Buddha

ARTWORK BY JEN FONTANILLA

Speaking negatively and thinking negative thoughts, both about ourselves and others, causes an increase in negative thoughts and behaviour. It's a self-perpetuating cycle and learning how to turn these thoughts on their head is key to overcoming low mood.

Negative Beliefs

Negative beliefs about yourself are debilitating in the worst way, because they are so easy to believe. And the more you tell yourself something, the more ingrained that belief becomes in your psyche. By challenging the negative beliefs you hold about yourself, you can acknowledge your positive qualities and boost your self-esteem. Here's a few ways to get started.

- Make a list of 3 things you like about yourself every night before bed. These can include personal attributes like kindness, physical attributes like: "I have a great nose," or something you did that day like: "I had quality time with my child today." Reflect on them and review them each week to remind yourself how awesome you really are.

- Stop treating yourself like crap. You heard me. Stop telling yourself you're a failure, a bad mother, a horrible friend. If you wouldn't say it to anyone else, stop saying it to yourself. Remember, your brain is smart, and the more you tell it something, the easier it becomes to see it as truth. Use affirmations ⌀ 1 to help you with this.

- Surround yourself with positive people. We talk about the impact this makes in Socialization. ⌀ 2

- When you achieve something, no matter how small, give yourself props for it! Celebrate your successes and enjoy your achievements. It's okay to be proud of yourself. I think there is this ingrained belief that if we're proud we are showing off, but the two are not mutually exclusive. It's not only okay to be proud, it is incredibly important for your self-esteem and self-worth!

You can't be both awesome and negative. Choose one.
-KAREN SALMANSOHM-

- Accept praise and compliments from others.

I have spent years trying to teach myself this. I always used to change the subject, push another person into the spotlight, or show the person all the things I *hadn't* achieved. Which is ridiculous! And I know I'm not alone in this behaviour. Many of us struggle with self-deprecation.

So much so that there have been studies done on it, and do you know what they found? When we self-deprecate, or put ourselves down, people are much less likely to continue complimenting us. Why? Because by exhibiting those negative behaviours, we tell others that we not only dislike being told nice things, but we are sending the signal that we are not worth praising.

So, it begins another vicious cycle. We feel unworthy, so we self-deprecate, because we self-deprecate people stop praising and complimenting us, and because they stop praising us, we feel even less worthy. So ridiculous, and yet so easy to fall into. Start small by saying 'Thank you' next time somebody compliments you, and then build up to holding an actual conversation about an achievement. It's hard, but so worthwhile!

- Another way to combat negative thoughts is to write them down and then tear up your paper and throw it away. Or even better - BURN THEM! I know this sounds juvenile, but research has proven that doing this signals your mind that those thoughts are worthless, and it needn't keep thinking about them. It's even being used in some types of therapy to help patients let go of negative thoughts.

- The reverse is also true. If you write down positive thoughts and put them in a safe place, your mind sees these as worthy of protection and consideration. Our brain only believes the information it is fed, and this means when we start providing it with positive thoughts, instead of reinforcing the negative ones, your brain, and you, start to believe them. [11]

Speaking negatively and thinking negative thoughts are both things that can mould your character and make a huge impact on your mood. But they can both also be altered, changed, and got rid of entirely. You're not stuck with them forever like some bad nose job.

Learn to start challenging negative thoughts. Why am I thinking this? What evidence do I have that it's true? Sort the fact from the fiction. Negative thoughts often come from beliefs we have held for most of our lives. Things that we think we cannot do, be, or say, may have been instilled in us as children and then reinforced by others, or even our own thinking over

---

[11] https://www.psychologicalscience.org/news/releases/bothered-by-negative-unwanted-thoughts-just-throw-them-away.html

the years. Because of this it can be harder for some people to overcome their negative thoughts than others. Harder, but not impossible. It is achievable!

The quality of your life is only as good as the quality of your thoughts, pure and simple. If you are constantly thinking miserable thoughts, then you will be miserable. If you are thinking and speaking negatively about your life, you will only see the negative. Try replacing your negative thoughts and words with positive ones. Practice gratitude - even if you've had a crap day. And find and focus on small positives. ✇ 3

So how do we go from smiling, happy children, to bitter, negative adults? And don't tell me that it's just reality that's set in, or that you are naturally pessimistic. 'Reality' isn't about how good or bad your life is, but about your perspective of it. Reality is defined as 'The state of things as they *actually* exist, as opposed to an idealistic idea of them.' So, reality is not negative or positive. It is simply reality. It is your viewpoint that puts the slant on each situation. Reality is like statistics. It can be viewed many different ways.

Here's an example.

Reality: Your train is delayed because a person threw themselves in front of the train

Viewpoint 1: My day was crap. I was already tired and then my train was delayed. The man on the seat next to me was taking up extra space, and the air conditioning was set too low.

Viewpoint 2: My day wasn't great, but it was better than some. I had a seat on the train while it was delayed, it didn't get too hot and sticky, and I am alive. And I got more time to read my book. Which is never bad!

Positive thinking helps you alter the way you view reality, and that has a huge impact on your mood.

How we see and react to everyday occurrences makes all the difference. For example: Looking at an object through water will distort how you see it. It's not a true representation. Once you take the object out of the water, however, you can see it more clearly. And that's all using a different perspective means. Simply viewing situations and thoughts without the distortion of negativity, sadness and other emotions. Technically the situation won't have changed at all, but your perspective, or understanding of it, will have.

> ☻ Errors in thinking, or cognitive distortions, are particularly effective at provoking or exacerbating symptoms of depression. It is still a bit ambiguous as to whether these distortions cause depression or depression brings out these distortions (after all, correlation does not equal causation!) but it is clear that they frequently go hand-in-hand.[12]

Negative Environment

Do you know anyone who you struggle to spend time with because you leave feeling drained? Why do you think this is? It's not usually because they are overly happy (although this can be exhausting when it's extreme too), but because in some way, shape, or form, they are negative.

Perhaps they love to gossip, pick, and poke at other people's lives. Perhaps they always find and focus on the negative aspects in their own lives, instead of the positive, and proceed

---

[12] https://positivepsychologyprogram.com/cognitive-distortions/

to tell you about them - at great length... Or perhaps they are often angry or irritable, or just a bit Eeyore-like.

Don't get me wrong, we are all guilty of these things at one point or another. I know I was particularly bad during my depression, and I must have been hard to be around. (Sorry, peeps). But our negative thoughts and feelings shouldn't define us. They shouldn't be the part of our character that people instantly see and think of when your name comes up. And if they are, then, honey, you've got some serious work to do. Because we weren't made to think and act negatively. We were born smiling! 🖊4

If you're discussing other people, be the one who always has something nice to say, no matter how small. If you are finding it really hard to be nice about someone, or think positively about them, stop for a moment. Ask yourself if you even need to spend time thinking or talking about them. My mum always used to say, "If you can't find something nice to say, don't say anything at all."

Instead of bitching about others or talking to people about the bad things happening in your life, try to talk about the things in your life that are good. You can still tell trusted friends and family members your troubles, and ask for advice, or vent to your friends. This can actually be very therapeutic and can help you identify and action solutions. Just don't make negative aspects the sum total of your conversation, every single time you catch up. Focus on the positive in your life and talk about it more than the negative!

Vent and then move on. 🖊5 If you're constantly revisiting the same old gripe, all you're doing is focusing your attention on the problem. And this is like looking at it through a magnifying glass. It only makes the problem bigger, and more present in your mind.

Think back to when you were a kid, and had scraped, bashed, or otherwise injured yourself enough to cause a hole somewhere on your body. Do you remember how hard it was to leave that scab alone when it started healing? Even when you knew you were doing more harm than good you still picked it.

Constantly focusing on, and talking about, the negative things in our lives is like picking a healing scab off over and over again. The wound never really gets a chance to heal. And the more you contemplate the injury, the less power you seem to have to stop yourself pulling off that scab!

In a weird way you admire your injury, you like the sympathy you get. You even revel in the pain of it. And it feels good when you're in the process of it. But when the scab comes off, you're back to square one. It hasn't improved the sore. In fact, it's made it worse, and increased the healing time.

And this is what thinking and talking negatively all the time does. It doesn't fix problems because there's no action linked to it. Negative thoughts and words, whether they are your own or someone else's, are toxic and should be avoided at all costs. So, you have 2 options.

1. Remove the negative thought, person, or environment from your life.

2. Pinpoint a solution and take actionable steps to resolve the issue. And then move on.

Personalizing

I used to have big problems with personalising everything. If a friend stopped calling or was never free to catch up, I immediately started thinking back to our last interaction. Clearly this was happening because of something I'd done, right? I must have said something or done something to offend them. I was in the wrong and I needed to rectify things.

Now while this may have been true occasionally, 99% of the time it was nothing at all. They were simply busy! Crazy, right? People being busy. But it wasn't just catching up with friends, I personalized every area of my life. It didn't matter the situation, I found some way to make it about me.

Which sounds really selfish when I put it like that. And it is, to a certain degree. But instead of stemming from an inflated self-importance, this way of personalizing everyone's actions stems from low self-esteem.

When you believe that you are unimportant, that you aren't smart, or good at your job, that you're a terrible mother, spouse, or friend, then it is incredibly easy to believe the worst in every situation. To believe everything bad is happening because of your shortcomings. And once you've created a scenario in your head it's incredibly hard to shake it, because:

YOUR BRAIN BELIEVES EVERYTHING YOU TELL IT!

I have found the best way to combat this is to take my negative thought and combat it with 3 'alternate truths,' 3 things that might be true other than the one I've latched onto. Take the example of the friend not calling above. My 3 alternate truths might be:

1. She is incredibly busy

2. She needs some personal time at the moment

3. She saw my text and responded in her head (we've all done this at some point!)

OR:

1. She's on holiday

2. She doesn't realise it's been so long (time really does fly)

3. She doesn't see catching up frequently as important as I do

Actually, this last one was an important insight for me because I tend to think everyone has the same values, priorities, and beliefs that I do, and of course that simply isn't true. People go through life in their own way, and how they do things may not always line up with how you think they should be. And that's fine. It's their life. Instead of trying to change them, work out how you can meet them halfway.

Telling myself 3 alternate 'truths' allowed me to come back to what was *actually* true, rather than getting worked up over the one 'truth' I'd created in my head. My friend has stopped calling. What can I do?

- I can reach out to see if she'd like to catch up

- See if she needs help with anything,

- Or just let her know I'm thinking of her

And you know what? 9 times out of 10 I'd end up ensconced on her lounge drinking tea and shooting the breeze, because guess what – she'd just been busy.

Alternate truths are essentially another way to diminish distortion and see the true picture. If you find yourself personalizing everything, then make sure you think of some alternate truths. They will change your whole perspective.

Past experiences, anger, sadness, negativity. They all distort. Think about how the symptoms of your low mood distort your vision. How do *you* react? Remember - bad things are always going to happen in our lives, but for every bad thing that happens, there are good ones too. We just have to look for and focus on them.⌀6 Not just every now and then, but consciously. Every day.

* * *

RECAP ✄

- Speaking and thinking negatively, both about ourselves and others, can cause an increase in negative thoughts and behaviour, mould your character, and have a huge impact on your mood. Learning how to combat this negativity is key to overcoming low mood.

- Negative thoughts and words are toxic, and negative beliefs about yourself are debilitating in the worst way, because they are so easy to believe. By challenging the negative thoughts you hold about yourself, you can acknowledge your positive qualities and boost your self-esteem.

- Learn to start challenging negative thoughts and sorting the fact from the fiction by asking yourself pointed questions. Why am I thinking this? What evidence do I have that it's true?

- Positive thinking helps you alter the way you view reality and provides you with distortion free perspective.

- Personalizing everyone's actions does not stem from selfishness but from low self-esteem. Combatting this with '3 alternate truths' is another great way to diminish distortion and see the real picture.

- The quality of your life is only as good as the quality of your thoughts.

ACTION STEPS ✎

Do now:

- See 'Affirmations' and pick one that suits you. Use this to start overwriting those negative thoughts with positive ones.

- Write down your concerns. Any and all of them. Go through them one by one and really focus on each thing. It is often easier to see a problem in context when it's written down. It becomes more real and we can focus on solutions rather than just having negativity rolling around our brains.

Plan to:

- Find ways to make other people's lives better, which in turn lifts you up. 🔗7

- Set specific times for thinking about negative situations. Our mind goes to bad places more often than we think, and having a specific time limits the amount we think negatively, while allowing our mind to see them as being dealt with. This helps break the cycle of negative thinking, and many people find they don't even want to think negatively in their specified time.

Work towards:

- Using the other hacks in *Choosing Happy* to overcome negativity.

- Giving yourself a telling off when you start having negative thoughts. Tell yourself to stop it, to move on, and to focus on something else. Sometimes just acknowledging the negative thought allows us to move past us.

LINKED TO

1. Say it Like You Mean It

2. Social Butterfly

3. Great Attitude

4. Smile – Your Face Won't Crack

5. Thinking Too Much About Crap You Shouldn't

6. Mind Your Mind

7. Give a Little

ABOVE ALL ELSE BE KIND

♪♫♪ ALL STAR — SMASH MOUTH ♪♫♪

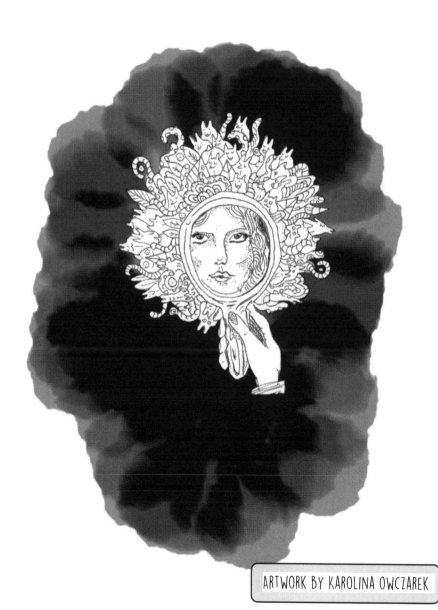

ARTWORK BY KAROLINA OWCZAREK

It seems silly to have to tell people to be kind to themselves, but unfortunately, we are our own worst enemies. We put everyone else first, we don't take care of our bodies, minds, or souls, and we are our own harshest critics. When we don't succeed at something we beat ourselves up over it, and when we do succeed we put it down to luck rather than skill or hard work.

> *"There's nothing you need to do, be, have, get, change, practice, or learn in order to be happy, loving, and whole."*
> -MICHAEL NEIL-

I mean, come on! Constantly telling ourselves we're a failure while not getting enough sleep, social interaction, good food, or exercise? It's a recipe for disaster! Positive emotions like joy, pride in ourselves, and contentment, on the other hand, not only feel amazing, but they also help us perform better, increase our resilience, and improve both our physical and mental health.

Perfection

I tend to get really worried that things are not perfect. When I launched my first creative endeavour - a small soft furnishings business, I spent months (ok, fine - years), making sure everything was just right before I presented it to the world.

Website, labels, tags, bags, fabrics, and the products themselves. I spent hundreds of hours on it. And I stressed! I worried I'd forgotten things. I worried nobody would like what I'd spent so long on. I stressed, and I worried, and I worked harder to combat this, which made me even more stressed and worried. It was a vicious cycle!

A close friend at the time also launched a small business making gorgeous children's clothes. She made a few, put them on Etsy and Facebook, and while they started selling she continued to build her brand, and get more products and all the little stuff together. I learnt a valuable lesson from her, and from many people since then. Done is better than perfect. You can fix and fiddle with things till the cows come home, but the reality is, most of the stuff you are stressing about can either wait 'til later or be skipped altogether.

We've all heard the expression 'don't sweat the small stuff,' but I had never really thought about it in line with perfectionism. What about 'get it done, get it going?' Heard that one? All these expressions tell us the same thing, if we actually listen. Things don't have to be perfect. Generally, the bulk of any task can be done in a small amount of time. It's all the little things that make a project or a chore drag out and cause stress and discontent.

"There are only two rules to life:
Rule #1. Don't sweat the small stuff.
Rule #2. It's all the small stuff."
-ROBERT ELIOT-

Life isn't made better by having a perfectly clean house, a perfect business model, or perfectly done nails. In fact, I feel this constant striving for perfection makes our lives more stressful, as we are always reaching for heights we generally never gain. This leads to a sense of failure, self-doubt, and sadness. I'm not saying you shouldn't try to excel in your work, in your studies, or in life in general. But there is a difference between aiming for greatness and clinging to perfection.

> (☻) Perfectionism may be the ultimate self-defeating behaviour. It turns people into slaves of success — but keeps them focused on failure, dooming them to a lifetime of doubt and depression. Perfectionists fear that if they give up perfectionism, they won't be good anymore at anything; they'll fall apart. In fact, perfectionism harms performance more than it helps. The worst thing about it is the belief that self-worth is contingent on performance — that if you don't do well, you're worthless. It's possible to escape that thinking.[13]

Many things in life just aren't important, when you get right down to it. **You need to ask yourself what matters most to you, is it a perfect life, or a joyous one?** Loosen your death grip on perfection, and it will loosen its grip on you.

Failure

Setting yourself achievable goals is a great way to boost your self-esteem.(✪) 1 But if you fail, don't beat yourself up! View mistakes and shortfalls as opportunities to learn. If you are failing, it means you are trying, and that in itself is to be applauded. Thomas Edison was famously quoted as saying: "I have not failed. I've just found 10,000 ways that won't work."

Now that takes some serious confidence in yourself. Edison knew he would figure it out eventually, and it didn't matter how often he failed, he kept on trying. If we never reach for great things we may never fail, but we also never succeed. Failure is an essential part of our lives, and instead of doing everything

---

[13] https://www.psychologytoday.com/us/articles/200803/pitfalls-perfectionism

we can to avoid it, we need to take a leaf from Edison's book and see it as just a stepping stone to success.

Failure helps mould us into the people we are, and when looked at from the perspective of Edison, is not a bad thing, but merely a learning curve. **Don't beat yourself up if you fail. Believe in yourself.** Have another crack, tackle the problem from a different angle, and above all, begin to see your failures as steps on the path to your eventual success, instead of something to be avoided at all costs.

Body Image

How long do you spend in front of the mirror before you go out, worrying if your hair looks nice, if your jeans make you look fat, or if you should wear the black heels or the tan ones? The sad truth is, it doesn't matter how you look, people are going to judge you regardless. The only way to be happy is to give yourself a break and start loving yourself. All the good bits, and all the bad bits too.

Don't let other people dictate your worth based on how you look, because the reality is, no one who is trying to live up to other people's expectations is happy. There is always one more thing they need to do, lose, or buy to make them 'perfect.'

Instead, wear clothes you're comfortable in and which you love. Buy new clothes based on your body type rather than the latest fashion. Ask the hairdresser which hair styles suit your face, rather than what's in vogue. Do the sports and activities you love regardless of how your body looks or works. You don't have to be perfect, you just have to be you!

Everyone is struggling with self-image, but the more comfortable you are in your own skin, the happier you will be. The happier you are with your body, and how you look, the more confident you'll become. And people who are confident are also much more attractive to others. It's true! Confidence is arguably one of the sexiest qualities in both men and women.

If people judge you for being yourself, then, honey, you need to find yourself some friends who don't. Because friendships and relationships are about loving a person for who they are, not how they look. And if it's a random stranger judging you, then who cares! You'll probably never see them again, and even if you do, their opinion shouldn't affect how you live and love your life and body. Often these people are speaking from a place of hurt and low self-esteem themselves. Yes, even the beautiful ones.

If you haven't already, check out a film called *Embrace* by Taryn Brumfitt. It is an insightful documentary about the global issue of body loathing. Its aim is to empower people to change the way we feel about ourselves, and our bodies, and is eye-opening. You can connect with Taryn on social media via the #bodyimagemovement, and she's also opened a course called 'Embrace You' online which teaches you practical strategies for how to embrace your body and your life.▶ A-maze-ing!

One of the biggest lies the documentary tackles is the belief that if we just lose 10 kilos, or tone our legs, or run 5 km, we will be happy. The reality is that there is always something else we aren't happy with. Just like buying objects can't make you happy, neither does having the perfect body. That stick-thin girl you envy probably hates that she has no curves. The fitness model probably wishes she could lose the tiny amount of fat on her back. (Taryn actually saw this first-hand during her stint as a fitness model).

The problem isn't with your body, the problem is what you think of it... and what you think of yourself

We all have things we don't like about ourselves, but my point is this. Even if your fairy godmother dropped out of a passing cloud and changed all those things, you would *still* find something you didn't like. Love it or hate it, your body is the only one you're going to get in this lifetime. And it is unique. No-one else has exactly the same shape, eyes, or hair. You are special. And you need to start celebrating how awesome you are. Because **regardless of whether you are fat, thin, tall, short, have crooked teeth, or wild hair, you are amazing!**

Belief

Believe in yourself! If you watch a presentation for a product and the producer seems unimpressed with it, would you buy it? No! And the same is true of people. If you don't believe in yourself, others will find it much harder to do so. Why do some people always get the job they're going for and others just as qualified don't? Because they have an unshakable belief in themselves. They know they have what it takes to succeed, and that belief shines out of them so much that others believe in them too!

Believing in yourself is something that happens when we give ourselves credit for jobs well done, ⌀ 2 when we celebrate our victories, and even our attempts. It comes when you focus on the good in yourself and visualize success. You may struggle. You may take two steps forward and one back, but that's okay! Take it one hour, one day, at a time. Persevere and keep believing in yourself, and you'll be amazed how fast you (and those around you) notice change.

Believing in yourself is like a drug. It lifts you up to dizzying heights and makes you feel capable of anything. And you know what? You are! Belief is one of the most powerful tools you can give yourself. If you believe something is possible, you will constantly search for ways to achieve it. Believe in yourself and your abilities, and tell the people around you, you believe in them too. Sometimes we need a little help seeing the greatness in ourselves.

Above all else, be kind. Not just to others, but to yourself.

* * *

RECAP 📌

- Positive emotions like joy, pride in ourselves and contentment help us perform better, increase our resilience, and improve both our physical and mental health.

- Things don't have to be perfect. In fact, constantly striving for perfection makes our lives more stressful. Ask yourself what matters most to you. Is it a perfect life, or a joyous one?

- Failure helps mould us into the people we are and should be viewed merely as a learning curve. If you're failing it means you're trying, and that in itself should be applauded.

- Don't let other people dictate your worth based on how you look. The only way to be happy is to start loving your body for what it can do, how it supports you, for the person it makes you, and to be comfortable in your own skin.

- Believe in yourself and your abilities and above all else, be kind. To others, and to yourself.

ACTION STEPS ✎

Do now:

- Make a list of *at least* 3 things you like about yourself.

Plan to:

- Ask a trusted friend or colleague (or several)! to tell you what they think your real strengths are. Remind yourself of these strengths when you're feeling less than awesome.

- Be as kind to yourself as you are to others.

- See your mistakes as opportunities to learn.

- Notice things you do well, however small.

- Celebrate your achievements

Work towards:

- Learning to love yourself for who you are right now.

- Believing in yourself

LINKED TO ⊘

1. Aim for the Stars

2. A Positive Spin on Negative Thoughts

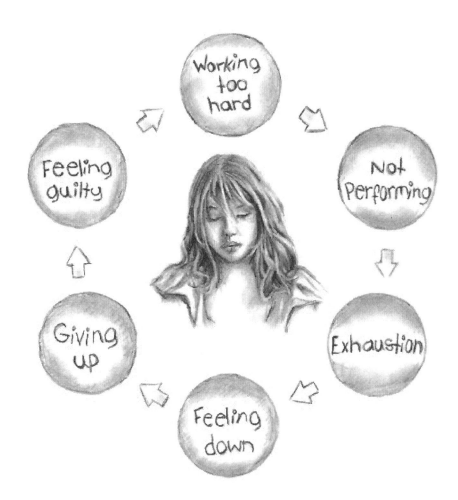

ARTWORK BY CRAIG DAWSON

ROUTINE

ROUTINES. I LIKE TO THINK OF THEM AS 'TO DO' LISTS WITHOUT THE LIST. THEY ALLOW YOU TO TAKE CHARGE OF YOUR DAY, COMPLETE TASKS, GROW GOOD HABITS, BUILD SKILLS AND KNOWLEDGE, AND MAKE THE MOST OUT OF LIFE BY PRIORITIZING WHAT IS IMPORTANT.

JUST MAKE SURE THAT YOU SET YOUR ROUTINE UP WITH THINGS THAT WORK FOR YOU, NOT FOR OTHER PEOPLE.

ROUTINELY AMAZING
♪♫♪ UPTOWN FUNK — MARK RONSON FT BRUNO MARS ♪♫♪

"Routine is not a prison, but the way to freedom from time."
- MAY SARTON -

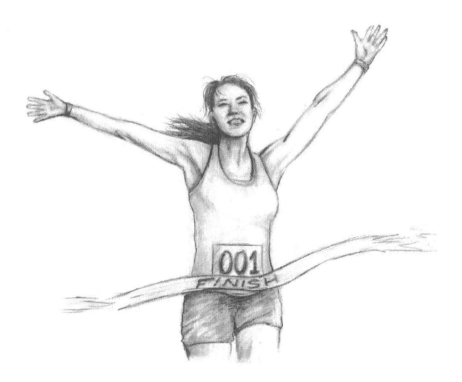

ARTWORK BY CRAIG DAWSON

Routine or rut? Rut or routine?

Is there even any difference? Yes, I think so. Routines are enjoyable and useful habits that, while performed repetitively, can still change and grow to include other things. Generally, with a rut you stagnate. A rut is just a routine you repeat because you can't be bothered to change it, or you think you shouldn't. These routines quickly become stifling and boring, and excuse the drama, crush your spirit. Hence the name 'rut.'

Often, it comes down to perception. If we tell ourselves we're in a rut, then all we'll see are the restrictions. If we see our routine as something that is benefiting us, then we will probably continue to enjoy the routine because we value it in some way, shape, or form. Routines only become ruts in our minds when they stop being useful and enjoyable and start becoming something we do *only* because it is habit.

Many people don't like having set routines because they see them as lead weights to creativity, spontaneity, and freedom. But a good routine is actually something that can give you more time to be creative, freedom to enjoy life, and can be altered or grown so that life is never boring.

So how do we form good habits and routines, without them becoming ruts? First you need to know what your goals are. 🔗 1 Once you know your goals you need to prioritize them, along with everything else life throws at you. 🔗 2

Finally, you can set up routines to make your goals and priorities happen. A good routine helps you make time for the important things, and ensures your life runs smoothly - without tying you down.

One of the best things I've learnt about building a routine is the magic 90-minute principal. You work for 90-minute chunks, and then alternate what you're doing so your brain gets a break. Why?

"The basic understanding is that our human minds can focus on any given task for 90-120 minutes. Afterwards, a 20-30-minute break is required for us to get the renewal to achieve high performance for our next task again. Instead of thinking what can I get done in my day, think about what you can get done in 90 minutes." [14]

In other words, stop multitasking, eliminate distractions, and just crack on for 90 minutes of awesome. Having that added deadline also increases the importance in your mind of getting it finished fast. Even with work, school runs, and other life commitments, you can still split your day into several 90-minute chunks to achieve more.

Successful people usually have incredible routines. And they don't have them because they have time. They have time because they have routines! They make their routines work for their lives rather than trying to fit their lives to a pre-set routine. Some take naps in the middle of the day and work late at night or in the wee hours of the morning. It's not something

[14] https://blog.bufferapp.com/optimal-work-time-how-long-should-we-work-every-day-the-science-of-mental-strength

that many of us could do, but it works for them, and that's what crafting a great routine is all about![15]

Sometimes I feel like my life is not my own because there are so many things pulling me in a multitude of directions. A routine gives your life structure and a sense of ownership. It helps you use your time well, even with life's other demands.

A morning routine is especially helpful, I find, because you don't have to decide what to do with your day. You know exactly what you're doing. It's already decided. This stops a lot of 'phaffing,' and fart-arsing around. Not only does this allow you to get straight into the day, it makes the day *yours*.

When you have a routine in place you also expend a lot less energy. You don't need to rely on motivation and willpower to get jobs done, you just do them because that's what's in place. This means that when you do need willpower to complete a task, it is not totally depleted. Willpower, like anything else, has a finite limit.

A good routine is kind of like cruise control. You just set and forget it, and expend far less energy in doing so, even though the distance is the same. Think of it like learning to run. You start off by running one lamppost and walking one. Then you start to run two lampposts and walk one, and so on, until you can run consistently. Routines are the same. They allow you to begin with small habits, and then build them into massive change. "From little things, big things grow."

Think back to the running analogy again. Every day you run, especially when you do it consistently, you get better at it. The same is true for things you add to your routine. You may be terrible at yoga when you first add it into your mornings, but

---

[15] https://blog.bufferapp.com/the-daily-routines-of-famous-entrepreneurs-and-how-to-design-your-own-master-routine

when you're doing something consistently every day, it soon becomes second nature. Routines are a great way to build existing skills or develop new ones.

Do you remember in "Rumination" we talked about your brain, and how it made pathways? 🔗 3 The more you used them, the more ingrained they got? Well, habits are the same. Apparently, we never really lose our old habits, they just get pushed into the background. How far back depends on how long we've been doing their replacements. Often our bad habits are so ingrained that without a routine we just revert back to them at any chance we get. Routines help us form new habits, and by doing them every day, ensure that we overwrite those old habit pathways with new, more positive ones.

When we follow a routine we not only make better use of our day, and implement good habits, we lift our mood through a sense of accomplishment and completion. We get a buzz out of charging through our morning and knowing we have succeeded in something! That, to me, is priceless because so often I get to the end of a very busy day and feel like I've achieved nothing. It's just been a slog.

> 😷 Routine adds elements of habit and rhythm into your daily life. Our bodies tend to function better when eating, sleeping, and exercise patterns are set to a regular schedule. Our minds also rely on patterns and routine. Because our brains have so much to process, they depend on habits to regulate daily processes.[16]

Routines also offer the reward of more time. I don't know about you, but there never seems to be enough hours in my day!

---

[16] http://mentalhealthcenter.org/boring-self-care-importance-routines/

Having a routine helps you get through a lot more, leaving you time for things you could never squeeze in before. That alone makes me love my routine.

So, what should you include in your routine? This is different for every person depending on how many hours you have available and what is important to you. Focus on those things that increase your mood, your perspective on life, and your growth, and go from there.

Do you want to write a book? Build writing into your day. Do you want to learn judo? Make judo lessons a part of your routine. Do you want to pursue a new career, build stronger friendships, start a business, learn to cook or craft? All these things can be worked on in your routine.

Here's some of the more common ones:

- **Exercise.** This is something we so often neglect or try to squeeze in at the last minute, and yet it is one of the most important things for you both mentally and physically. As a society, we sit far more than ever, so even if it's only walking to work or the shops, make it happen! ⊘4

- **Family.** Did you know we are spending more time than ever before with our children? And yet, how often do we sit down and focus all our attention on just one member of our family? Without TV, without phones, without jobs, dinner, or other distractions? Just you, and them. Building bonds with family members is vitally important and takes just a few quality minutes a day.

- **Friends.** Make sure catching up with friends, even briefly, is a part of your day-to-day life. ⊘5

- **Learning.** Learning new skills and gaining knowledge is one of the things that encourages us to flourish and grow as individuals. If you want to learn a language, a skill set, or gain knowledge in a particular area, a routine can help. 🖉6

- **Chores.** Work out what has to be done each week - only what's important - and set a particular day for it. I do all my chores and errands one day, all my cleaning on another, and have my third 'free day' set aside for myself and my friends.

Use this list to develop a routine for your whole week - that includes your weekends too! Remember, a routine doesn't have to be work related or be about getting the most done possible. It is about utilizing your day to incorporate things *you* want to achieve in your life, and make them a habit, even if your routine revolves solely around relaxing.

Your routine doesn't have to be the same every day either. In fact, many people find that setting specific tasks for specific days works better for them. You can 'theme' your days for chores, work, friends, or 'you' time, and still be assured that you are getting done what needs to be done.

Keeping your routine flexible also means you can be spontaneous, something that's really important. This means you won't feel restricted. Using those 90-minute blocks we talked about is a great way to keep your routine flexible. Instead of writing an hour by hour routine you can just add several 90-minute blocks and keep the rest flexi. Your routine should be a help, not a hindrance.

You can even use apps like 'Coach.Me' to help you build positive change and routine. This free iPhone and Android app lets you choose habits you want to include in your life and set reminders to do them. You can tick when you've done something and track your momentum through graphs over both weeks and months. It also has a great online community that provides encouragement and healthy peer pressure. Did I mention all this was free?

Look at the best time of day for each thing in your routine. Everybody naturally has peaks and lows in their energy, and some things are just easier to accomplish at certain times of the day. Science has shown that we actually do our best creative work when we're tired, so leave anything creative 'til after your more analytical work.

Many countries still have a siesta in the afternoon as this is generally when our energy is the lowest, and those entrepreneurs we mentioned earlier who nap in the afternoon are doing a similar thing. Having just a 20 minute 'nana nap' can increase your energy and focus and mean you actually get more done in your day than if you'd just pushed through. Some expert nappers can even nod off on their desks at work! If napping just isn't going to happen, then try something else relaxing in the early afternoon such as meditation, yoga, or sitting quietly with a cup of tea.

I am super focused first thing in the morning, so this is the best time for me to write. If I exercise in the middle of the day, this then gives me energy to do all my jobs before relaxing or creating in the evening. In theory. I'm always tweaking my routine as I find out what works best for me, and you will need to do the same. Don't just expect to get it right first time. Instead of avoiding change, invite it, so you can really narrow down what works best for you and your life.

Basically, routines disrupt bad habits, and replace them with good ones, while making the best use of the day, and building new skills and knowledge. Brilliant.

* * *

RECAP 📌

- A good routine ensures your life runs smoothly, can give you more time to be creative, and helps you make time for important things. It gives your life structure and a sense of ownership and helps you use your time well.

- A good routine can also be altered and grown to suit your changing life. A routine that doesn't allow change can quickly become a rut. A routine should always be a help, not a hinderance. Tweak your routine as you find out what works best.

- Routines are a great way to build existing skills or develop new ones. They're also great at helping us form new habits.

- There are many different ways to set up a routine. Try laying yours out in 90-minute chunks. These provide your brain with a deadline and increases the importance in your mind of getting your task finished fast. Switching tasks after 90 minutes also gives your brain a much-needed break. Or you could set specific tasks for specific days, creating 'themed' days.

- A routine doesn't have to be all work related or about getting as much done as possible. It is about disrupting bad habits, making the best use of the day, and building new skills and knowledge.

ACTION STEPS ✎

Do now:

- Write down everything you would like to include in your week.

- Look through *Choosing Happy* and use the chapters to help you decide what's important or have a brainstorming session. Just make sure the things you choose are those you *want* in your life, not those you *think* you should have!

- Use 90-minute time slots where possible to help you chunk through big jobs, give you a time frame, and keep your brain fresh and firing. Here are a few things you may like to include.

Plan to:

- Start eating a decent breakfast. A good breakfast can still be fast and easy and gives you a lot more energy and focus for the day ahead. ✪7

- Save creative work for when you're tired. Get the big, analytical jobs done while you're fresh.

- Set alarms to help you remember the things you planned while you're getting used to your routine.

- Change your routine. You'll discover what works and what doesn't as you begin using your routine. Don't be afraid to change it up!

Work towards:

- Having a routine in place that really works for you. Make sure it allows time for everything you need and want to do in life - not just that work nonsense.

- Track your habits to understand yourself better, and change your routine as needed.

- Adding new things into your routine so it doesn't stagnate, and so you grow and develop as a person.

LINKED TO

1. Aim for the Stars

2. Sort Your Crazy

3. Thinking Too Much About Crap You Shouldn't

4. Exercise Your Mind

5. Social Butterfly

6. Learning to Grow

7. Eat the Food!

SORT YOUR CRAZY

♪♫♪ BEST DAY OF MY LIFE — AMERICAN AUTHORS ♪♫♪

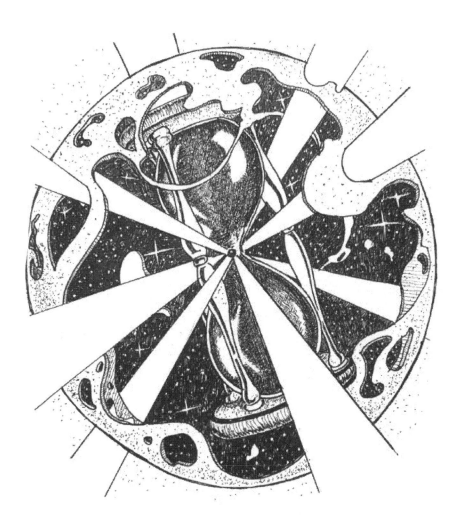

ARTWORK BY ASHWIN PILLAI

Prioritizing helps you put the things you value at the top of your list and teaches you how to view life with better perspective. Your family, your friends, your job, your health, travel, and yourself. It's easy to say on paper that we value our family first, but actively prioritizing what's important in your life helps you reflect those priorities in your actions, as well as your thoughts.

The key is not to prioritize what's on your schedule but to schedule your priorities.
-STEPHEN COVEY-

Often in life we end up doing all the little things, the 'minutiae' of life, the things we 'have' to get done, and neglecting the really important things.

Prioritizing the things we value most helps us do what makes us happy, instead of what we feel we have to get done. This is amazing! Because how often do we get to the end of the week and realise we haven't done a single thing we really wanted to, but got lots of 'stuff' done? Work, school runs, washing, dishes. These sorts of things are always there, they are the 'fillers' of life. It doesn't matter how often you do them, they are right back there the next day.

I'm not saying you should stop going to work or leave dirty dishes everywhere, but make sure you don't do these things exclusively. Do the important things first and do the dishes in the spare time rather than the other way around.

Let's look at it from a different angle. You have 2 hours in which to tidy the house before friends arrive for dinner that night. You are just tidying up the last thing when they walk in the door. Phew! Lucky you had two hours! Now, imagine you had decided to go for a run for an hour, leaving you only one hour to clean. What happens? You still get everything done as they walk in the door.

Why? When we have lots of time to do a task we don't do it with the energy or speed we do if we have limited time. On top of that, we 'fill' time with things that don't really need doing. Did the house need a dust? Yes, probably. Did it need a dust right then? Probably not. When we prioritize our lives, we put the big, important things first so that we make sure they are included in our day. Then we add the things we have to do, and lastly the 'fillers' if we have time.

> ☢ You must learn to detach your sense of satisfaction and accomplishment from the number of check marks you have on your to-do list at the end of the day. In my opinion, you've been more productive on a day in which you've crossed off one thing out of ten, if it was the most important task, rather than nine things, leaving the most important still undone. [17]

Often, we get this order arse about face. We start with all the little things, so we get them 'out of the way,' then we do the things that have to be done, and if we have time we include all those things we love and are important to us. We spend time with friends, we have dinner with the family, we exercise and enjoy our hobbies. I don't know about you, but when I die I want to look back and see a life filled with amazing experiences. I don't want to see loads of washing with only the occasional mountain bike ride!

---

[17] http://www.theproductivitypro.com/FeaturedArticles/article00017.htm

I'm sure you've all heard the story of the philosophy teacher who was lecturing on time management? Instead of just speaking to his class he conducted an experiment called the 'jar of life.'

He placed a large jar on his desk and began by adding big rocks to it until the class agreed it was 'filled.' He then added smaller pebbles, which filtered through the big rocks until the students once again agreed the jar was 'full.' The professor then went on to tip sand into the jar, which filled all the little spots between the rocks. Water was then poured into the jar until it was brimming. This he used as an analogy of life.

"You see," he told the class, "if we don't put all the larger stones in the jar first, we will never be able to fit all of them in later. If we give priority to the smaller things in life (pebbles & sand), our lives will be filled up with less important things, leaving little or no time for the things in our lives that really matter to us."

What the large stones are in your life is for you to decide. They might be health, family, friends, goals, travel, fighting for a cause, or simply taking time for yourself. Whatever your 'big stones' are, be sure to put them first in your 'Jar of Life,' or you may find you never have time for them. And these are the things that make life the incredible adventure it is!

The small things in life, the minutiae, are on repeat anyway. You do the dishes and they appear again. You clean the house and bam! It's dirty again. Lawns are mowed and the next minute the grass is waving around your feet. Do you want your life to just be a long stretch of 'keeping on top of things?' The big things in our lives, those 'large stones,' are the things that make us happy. They are the things we look back on with joy, remember when we need a boost, and look forward to with anticipation!

I've posted the top 5 regrets of the dying collated by Bronnie Ware ▶ below, not because I want you to think about dying, but because I want you to think about how you would live and what you would do with your day if you knew you were! What is important to you?

Top 5 Regrets of the Dying.

1. Not being true to yourself. Don't let the expectations of others get in the way of what makes you happy.

2. Spending too much time working. We can't take money with us, and we can't get back the years we wasted working instead of building relationships and enjoying life.

3. Leaving things unsaid. Trying to avoid conflict actually made for more stress and friendships that weren't as strong in the long run.

4. Not staying in touch with friends. Time constraints and not prioritizing friendships meant that people missed out on what could have been wonderful moments in their lives.

5. Not letting themselves be happy. The fear of what others think, their fear of change, and the comfort of the familiar stopped them from having fun and experiencing joy the way they could have.

The bottom line is this. **Don't just find time to do the things you love, make time. Because this is what life is really about. Living.** Prioritize the things in life that are important to you and do them first! You will still find the jobs get done, but without the filler and wasted time your days had previously.

Don't let other people dictate your life, and your happiness. Live your life like every day was your last, because one day it will be. Make them count! Put those big rocks first and don't just prioritize things in your thoughts, but in your actions.

Now, back away from the washing machine and go play with your child or enjoy a walk with a friend. Because this is your life. And you only get one.

* * *

RECAP 📌

- Prioritizing helps you put the things you value at the top of your list and teaches you how to view life with better perspective.

- Often in life we end up doing all the minutiae of life because they 'have' to be done, neglecting the truly important things. And yet it is those big things we neglect that make us happy and give us a sense of satisfaction and accomplishment.

- How would you live and what would you do with your day if you knew you were dying? These are the things you should be making time for every day.

- It's up to you to not just find time, but to make time for the things that are important to you.

ACTION STEPS ✏️

Do now:

- Write a list of everything that's important to you in your life. Brainstorm for 10 minutes at the minimum and write down everything that comes into your head, no matter how small or stupid sounding!

- Order your list into 'Rocks,' 'Pebbles,' 'Sand,' and 'Water.' Or most important to least important if you want to be boring.

- Think of at least 3 ways you can start prioritizing the things that are most important to you. Hint: a great way to start is by creating a routine. ⊘1

Plan to:

- Each morning I want you to wake up and decide on *one* thing you want to do that day. Not what you need to get done, but one thing that's important to you. One of your big rocks. Add this to your goals list for the day and prioritize it.

- Reflect on your day every night and make sure you're including the things you love. Benjamin Franklin had it right. He used to ask himself every morning, "What good shall I do this day?" This was something that was important to him. In the evening, he would reflect on his day and say, "What good have I done today?" What a dude!

Work towards:

- Having all your ducks in a row. Or your landscaping materials if you want to continue the rock analogy. Whatever. Get your priorities happening on a daily basis and make it such a habit that you don't even think twice about whether you play a board game with your kid or sweep the floor. (It's a no-brainer, really, isn't it?)

LINKED TO ⊘

1. Routinely Amazing

AIM FOR THE STARS
♪♫♪ ON TOP OF THE WORLD — IMAGINE DRAGONS ♪♫♪

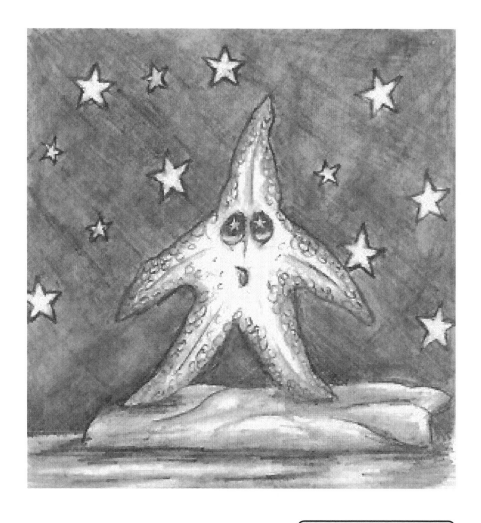

ARTWORK BY CRAIG DAWSON

Making goals for our future is an important way to ensure our present is what we'd like it to be. What do I mean? Here's a real-life example for you.

My sister-in-law has been thinking about quitting her job as a teacher for a while. It will be a massive loss to the world because she is awesome at it, but it is also stressful and exhausting. We really don't give teachers enough kudos - they do an incredible job! She looked at her present happiness and realised that the things she loved doing, she didn't have the time or energy for.

So, she created some future goals around making sure this changed. She set up a plan for quitting her job. She told her friends (accountability), she wrote her CV, she restructured her mortgage, tidied her spare room so she could rent it out, and made several contingency plans.

She had thought about quitting before but had never been able to see how it would work. By setting herself goals, it has now become achievable. Her *now* wasn't what she wanted, so she made plans she could work towards to make sure her *future now* was. A real life *Choosing Happy*.

If we can't look forward and see something exciting, challenging, or enticing waiting for us in our future, then it's hard to be inspired. And if we're not looking forward, and the present isn't how we really want it to be, then all we're left with is looking back. And let's just say it's not usually the good things we focus on when we start looking backwards.

Much of the stress we feel in our lives is caused by never enjoying the moment. By constantly looking forward to the next 5 or 10 things that have to be done. The idea of setting goals is not to ignore or gloss over the present, but to ensure the path you're on is taking you where you want to be in your future. Goals work in the same way that a map does. They show you what path to take but don't diminish your enjoyment of that path. Goals are simply a way of pointing you in the right direction.

The goals you set should be based on your happiness in the present. What would make you happier now? What would you change in your life if you could? What changes do you need to make to achieve this? These are the things you set goals for. I'm not talking about material goals like 'I want to be a millionaire in 10 years,' or 'I want to own a Dodge Challenger in 5' (drool...). I'm talking about happiness goals.

You don't have to have something as big as quitting your job on the horizon. Even small changes in our everyday routine can be things to look forward to. The old adage "a change is as good as a break" is as true now as it was when it was coined. Perhaps you want to change how much time you spend with family, try one new recipe a week, or say hello to that person you keep seeing on the train. As we discuss in Learning to Grow 1, the very act of anticipating and participating in new things increases our happiness.

Goals are a fabulous way to motivate us and ensure the things that make us happy become a reality. They are also an integral part of our ability to grow and change as a person. Without goals we wander aimlessly and don't achieve nearly as much in life. So, take the first step and set yourself some goals. For the day, the month, and the year. And even 5 and 10 years down the track. Make your goals challenging enough to excite you, while also being achievable.

Your goals could be as small as drinking more water each day, to something much larger like starting your own company. You could include travel goals, learning to juggle, or speak a new language. It doesn't matter what your goals are, as long as they are happiness goals. Things that will improve your life. Make sure whatever you choose are things that you want for yourself - not dictated by or for others. These are *your* life goals, not theirs!

By setting yourself clear, concise goals, you are creating a road map to the future you want to live. You may not make it to where you're going, you might get side-tracked enjoying the path along the way, but the great thing is, even if you don't achieve all your goals, your mood is boosted simply by having a sense of purpose.

Ingvar Kamprad, who was the founder of IKEA (and one of the world's richest men), has been quoted as saying:

"Happiness is not reaching your goal, happiness is being on the way. So, let's talk about goals, and how they can not only help you achieve your ideals, but give you a bright, happy future to look forward to."
-INGVAR KAMPRAD-

Daily goals

Small goals are just as important as big ones because they provide instant gratification. Had coffee with a friend? Check. Made your bed? Check. Small goals allow you to streamline and enjoy your life, without the long wait between thinking of a goal and completing it.

I am a list girl. I love lists. I write them for everything. (I also add things to my list I've already done that day just so I can cross them off...) The problem with writing massive lists is that we never seem to get to the end of them. And that can be crushing and incredibly stressful. It feels like we've been busy all day but haven't actually achieved anything! Feeling overwhelmed and incompetent? I used to all the time, so I tried to stop writing lists. But then I used to feel like I'd forgotten something important, and I'd get that annoying niggling feeling all day.

So, I started writing lists again, but now I write them a little differently. I still write a big list of 'to do's,' but I no longer set out to cross as many things off the list as I can each day while constantly adding more. Now I do a daily 'top 3.' And it is working fabulously. Here's how I do it:

I get everything out of my head and onto my 'to do' list. Then I look through my list and pick out the top 3 things that I really want or need to get done that day. Just three. No more, no less. I try to pick a combination of big and small things, while also taking into account how much free time I have that day. If it's a day I normally buy groceries, that becomes the first item on my list. Then I might want to get some writing done, which becomes number two. Then exercise or catching up with a friend would be number three.

For me, I know that socialization, exercise, and writing are all incredibly important for my mental wellbeing. And yet they are all things I never used to make time for, because I had an endless list of jobs that 'had' to be done. By writing them into my daily goals they become as important in my mind as they should be. Not only do I still get chores done, but I am in a much happier place for having a more balanced life. ✐ 2

Lists can be excellent. They help remind you what needs to be done and show you how you're progressing, if you use them right. I try to do one big house chore, one work task, and one personal activity each day. Your top three will be made up of things that are important to you. Just make sure that your lists are not all work related but are a good mix of tasks and personal goals.

Future goals

Choosing realistic goals gives our lives direction, and brings a sense of accomplishment and satisfaction when we achieve them. But how do you make sure that the goals you're setting are meaningful, achievable, and sustainable?

Well, start by writing down things that are important (or meaningful) to you, and your vision for the future. There is no point including things we think we should do but don't really want to. How much motivation are you going to have to complete those kinds of goals? Meaningful goals are those that make us excited just thinking about them!

"My interest in life comes from setting myself huge, apparently unachievable challenges and trying to rise above them... from the perspective of wanting to live life to the full, I felt that I had to attempt it."
-SIR RICHARD BRANSON-

Not all goals have to be achievable right away. In fact, **setting far off, wild goals that we don't really know if we can achieve is actually a great idea.** Why? Because it gives us something to aim for. We may not make it all the way, but setting outlandish goals helps show us what we're really capable of and extends our abilities far more than just working towards easy goals. This in turn helps boost our sense of self-worth and our confidence.

If you don't know how to tackle a large goal, break it down into small chunks and start by completing one step at a time, like a ladder. Looking at a large goal in small parts is nowhere near as overwhelming, and also helps you track your progress, as you can mark off each small step on your way.

Successful business people know what they want out of life. They have goals, and with these goals they have a clear vision of the future that they can then pursue. And individuals should be no different. Set goals. Take steps towards making them happen. Include both personal goals and work-related goals. They are both part of your life.

⊛ Sir Richard Branson has a lot to say about goals, and for good reason. He started his first business venture at the ripe old age of 16, and is the founder of the Virgin Group, which currently controls over 400 companies! He wasn't abnormally smart, in fact he suffered from dyslexia and got poor school grades, but he had a vision for his future and he set out to make it happen.

It can be incredibly hard to keep chasing far off goals if you never see any progress. Working your future goals into your daily goals list can help you track progress, stay excited, and also helps ensure that your goals are sustainable long term.

Making your goals work

Instead of writing a massive list of goals and trying to make all of them happen at once, pick *one* goal you're aiming for, and do just *one* thing to get started. Then work out what the next few steps are to achieve that goal and work them into your daily routine.

Long term goals often take quite a bit of time for a reason. Money, experience, or life obstacles have to be sorted first, so set a long-term goal in motion and then simultaneously work on short-term ones. Not only does this mean you are achieving more, but you don't get bored and give up.

Share your goals with others. It is so much harder to back out of a goal if people are holding you accountable, or even asking you how you're going. Tell at least 3 people about a goal that is really important to you this year, or if you're feeling really brave, broadcast it on social media! I did this with my "Greatest Shave" campaign because I was scared if I didn't I'd back out of it!

Make your goals measurable so you can see how you're going. Sometimes we look back and feel like we've done a lot of hard yards without any results. When I wrote my first book I was advised to write down a few goals that I wanted to meet once published. And I am so glad I did! I was already feeling incredibly overwhelmed just putting my creative work in the public eye, and then to feel like I wasn't achieving anything was crushing.

So, when I dragged out my list of expectations and found that I had met or exceeded, not just some, but all of them, I was pretty surprised! It is human nature to achieve something and instantly want more (this is why 'having' doesn't make you happy). So, it is incredibly important to not only know what you *want* to achieve, but to write it down so you can measure your achievements accurately.

Celebrate your successes! One of the things that makes achieving goals so much fun is the sense of satisfaction we get. Don't rush onto the next goal as soon as you've achieved one. Get excited! Celebrate! Be proud of yourself! And *then* write some new goals.

* * *

RECAP ✦

- Goals are a fabulous way to motivate us. And making goals for our future is an important way to ensure our present is what we'd like it to be. If we can't look forward and be excited, challenged, or enticed then it's hard to be inspired.

- The idea of setting goals is not to ignore or gloss over the present, but to ensure the path you're on is taking you where you want to be in the future.

- Not all goals are achievable right away, but it doesn't matter! Your mood is boosted simply by having a sense of purpose. And setting outlandish goals shows us what we are capable of and extends our abilities. They also boost our self-worth and self-confidence. Break large goals into bite sized pieces to make them easier to tackle.

- Small goals are important too as they provide instant gratification and encourage us to keep going.

- Writing lists can be a great way of goal setting for the day. If you do them right. Put everything in your head onto a 'to do' list. Then pick ONLY 3 things to complete that day.

- Make sure your goals are meaningful to YOU.

ACTION STEPS ✎

Do now:

- Write down every idea, dream, and plan you have for the future. Nothing is too small, too large, or too ridiculous. If it's important to you, write it down! You can write bullet pointed lists, keep a notebook of ideas, or even use pictures to create a visual ideas list. What calls to you?

- Choose one goal that you can complete in the time you have left today and go do it! It feels so amazing ticking things off, and it may help give you the boost you need to set more complex goals.

Plan to:

- Make a list of goals you'd like to achieve this week. Some small, some big. And again, make sure they are things *you* want to achieve. Each day pick the top three things you'd like to get done. Never roll jobs over into the following day. If you didn't complete something, put it back onto your big list, and pick a fresh three for the new day. This might include the previous day's goals, it might not. Every day is different, and the only thing we achieve by rolling over goals is that feeling of being swamped and stressed. And that is exactly what we're trying to avoid!

- Reflect on your goals. Don't just set and forget them. This is a sure way to never complete them. Every week, look at the goals you had set and see how you went. Did you achieve them? What could you do differently next week? Are you on your way to achieving other goals?

- Tell people. Share your joy and excitement about a goal you're aiming for on social media or with friends and family. Not only does this increase your happiness, it holds you accountable, and encourages you to complete your goal.

- Celebrate your successes!! If you've posted your goals on social media, update people. You'll be surprised at the responses. People love to celebrate others' successes, especially if you are genuinely happy about achieving something, rather than just showing off. If we never celebrate our wins, it becomes harder and harder to have any kind of enthusiasm for completing goals. You've done well. Enjoy!

Work towards:

- A large life goal. Nothing is quite so pleasurable as working towards something you never thought would happen. Break it down into small steps. Do one thing this week to start working towards your big, awesome goal.

LINKED TO 🔗

1. Learning to Grow

2. Sort Your Crazy

GET OUT OF BED YOU DAISY HEAD
♪♫♪ WAKE ME UP — AVICII ♪♫♪

I love the smell of possibility in the morning.

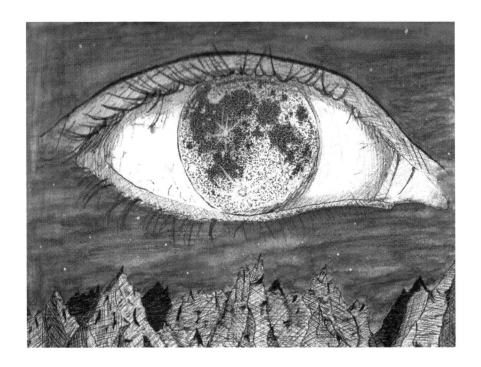

ARTWORK BY BEN DAVID PUGH

One routine we should all have is a morning routine. People are most productive when they first wake up, and setting a routine helps you start the day right and sets the tone for the rest of the day. It's one of the most powerful things you can do.

Everyone's morning routine will be different because we all have very different lives. Some people aren't morning people at all, and struggle to function first thing. Others don't have much time in the morning because they leave early for work or are woken to a small child asking you to admire their latest artwork.

Work, exercise, children, sleep! It doesn't matter what dominates your morning, a routine can help. Aim for at least a half hour morning routine, with as much of it done as possible without interruption.

I hear you laughing, mums around the world. Uninterrupted time. That's hilarious! Seriously though. This could be the only time of the day where you get to stop, think, discover, and relax your body and mind without a hundred other things happening. Do what you have to, to carve out time for yourself first thing. Get up half an hour earlier, lock yourself in the bathroom, escape to the garage, or down to the park. Find something that works for you and is sustainable.

> ☻ "What I have found over and over again is that early risers are the kinds of people who make healthier choices. They are more likely to exercise in the morning, eat a healthy breakfast, and make time for reading, yoga, prayer, meditation, or other healthy and fulfilling habits." -JEFF SANDERS-

I cannot stress enough how important making time for yourself is first thing in the morning. The start of the day often sets the pace and the emotional state for the rest of the day. Do you start each day rushing, annoyed, and overwhelmed? How much of a difference do you think it would make if you started your day feeling relaxed, refreshed and prepared for whatever life threw at you? I know from personal experience that if I start my day well, it is far easier to stay on that track. And vice versa.

Ever notice how when one bad thing happens in the morning the rest of your day seems to be full of them? It may not necessarily have any more negative aspects than any other day, but when our minds and bodies are stressed we tend to notice and react to things differently, creating a negative feel, or taint to the day 🔎 1. Starting the day positively ▶ can really help combat this effect.

Below you'll find a list of things that you could include in your morning routine. Each one has a time listed or 'creates time.' These are just a guide to help you see what you can fit into your morning routine. I would suggest picking at least one item from each category, and ensuring you are realistic.

If you normally have 10 minutes to get ready, don't assume that having a routine is going to give you a spare hour. Mornings are usually busy times, but if you try to wake up a bit earlier than usual or do preparation the previous day to make your mornings are freer, then you will have more time for personal things such as goal setting, meditation, and affirmations.

Giving yourself a calm, quiet morning helps create energy and the right mindset to tackle challenges throughout the day. Ideally, everyone should have been awake for an hour and a half before walking out the door, but this isn't realistic for many people. So, do what you can, and do it consistently, and you'll see huge changes.

Environment

- Wake up with the sun and let the natural light in. The sun controls the body's circadian rhythm. This is the thing that makes your energy levels rise and dip. Waking up with the sun helps your rhythm stay balanced so you can manage your energy levels better. Getting up with the sun also gives us more time and helps us feel more rested and more productive. Science has even proven that waking up early benefits our moods.

Of course, there's always that one person... my editor swears if she's caught in a sunbeam and not moving she gets sleepy regardless of how much sleep she's had! She's one of 17% of the population who actually function better at night[18]. If this is you, then try waking up to a sunrise lamp. Sunrise lamps mimic a natural sunrise, so you can have the same great effects, but at a time that suits you and your routine. This is also great for those winter months when the sun rises well after when you need to be up.

"Sunlight is the most potent stimulant that gives energy and improves your mood."[19]

Remember, the more natural light you're exposed to in the morning, the easier it will be for you to not only

---

[18] https://www.livescience.com/16334-night-owls-early-birds-sleep-cycles.html
[19] Alcibiades J. Rodriguez, MD, assistant professor, Department of Neurology, NYU Langone Comprehensive Epilepsy Centre-Sleep Centre

wake up but get out of bed. And if you can't get morning sun, make sure you grab some later in the day. Your body needs it! 🖉 2 **Creates time**

- Have the space where you go to meditate or exercise free of clutter and distractions. This means you can get straight into your routine without being interrupted by other things. **Creates time**

- Be prepared the night before so you're not rushing in the morning. Lay out your exercise clothes and/or work clothes. Organise breakfasts and lunches. Have work and school bags packed and waiting by the door. **Creates time**

Body

- Rehydrate. Your body is most dehydrated first thing in the morning. Rehydrate with a glass of warm lemon water. This helps you wake up faster, lubricates your bowels, and aids digestion. You can even add mint. It's a natural stimulant and increases mental alertness. Have your morning supplements or probiotics with it. **Time - 5 mins**

- Have a green smoothie. Green and antioxidant smoothies boost energy, provide fibre, minerals, and phytonutrients. They are easy to digest because the plant walls have been broken down from blending and are pure nutrition. **Time - 10 minutes**

- Eat a nutritious breakfast. Good carbohydrates like fruit and whole grains help fuel your body and brain and provide fibre. 🖉 3 Add protein and healthy fats to slow digestion and help you feel 'full.' Yum! **Time - 20 minutes**

- Scrape your tongue and clean your teeth. Not only does this get rid of morning breath, it helps keep your teeth and gums healthy and gets rid of toxins, and it aids wakefulness, which is always welcome first thing. **Time - 5 mins**

- Dry brush your body. This improves circulation, which helps invigorate you, sloughs off dead skin cells, and leaves your skin feeling smoother. (It also warms me up, which is great because I can be a cold fish first thing.) **Time - 10 minutes**

- Palming. Rub your palms. Place them gently on closed eyelids so the cups of the hand cover the eyelids. There should be no pressure. Soothes the eyes and rests the mind. Can be done in conjunction with meditation ◎ 4. **Time - 1-10 mins**

Mind

- Listen to uplifting music. Helps start the day with a great mindset. Soothing music for de-stressing, or energetic for getting into action. **Time- 5-10 mins**

- Meditate, pray, or journal for a few minutes. Helps clear and calm your mind and increases creativity and memory. You can also use a meditation app, or guided meditation. **Time - 10 mins**

- Feed your mind with positive thoughts first thing. This will impact the rest of your day. It doesn't matter if these thoughts are from reading the Bible, the Koran, or a motivational book, from listening to an audiobook or a podcast, or reviewing thoughts from a positivity jar or your vision board. You can even just sit quietly and think about positive things in your past, present, and future. It doesn't matter, as long as they are positive. **Time - 5 minutes**

- Smile at yourself in the mirror for 30 seconds. This ridiculously simple hack helps boost your self-esteem and starts your day with positivity🔗5. **Time - 1 minute**

- Recite your affirmations🔗6. Do this together with smiling in the mirror. **Time - 1 minute**

Exercise

- Stretch baby, stretch! Do a stretching routine such as yoga to help wake up your muscles. Yoga increases lung capacity. Helps with memory, relieves anxiety, and lowers the risk of heart disease - among other things! **Time - 10 minutes**

- Rebound 100 times. This helps keep you energized without sugar or caffeine. What the! It also firms up your body, clears your sinuses, and increases those creative juices. **Time - 5 minutes**

- Have a jam session. Fire up your favourite song and dance to it. Sing along. Guaranteed to put you in a happy, energized mood. **Time - 5 minutes**

- Workout and break a sweat. (see "Exercise" for more how's and why's🔗7) **Time - 30 minutes**

Future

- Remind yourself of the 'why.' Why am I doing this? What do I love about my life? If today was my last day on earth, what would I do? What would I regret? This provides clarity on what's important and helps you focus. **Time - 5 minutes**

- Write out your top 3 goals for the day. This builds confidence and helps prioritize ↪ 8. **Time - 5 minutes**

- Review your future goals. This helps remind yourself of what's important. **Time - 5 minutes**

Connection

- Text something encouraging to a friend or leave a note. Brightening someone else's day also improves your own happiness and outlook on life ↪ 9. **Time - 5 minutes**

- Write part of a letter or email. This helps you stay in touch with friends and family and alleviates loneliness ↪ 10. **Time - 5 minutes**

- Be accountable to someone. Connect with like-minded people on an online group or forum, or with friends and family in person or through technology. Track your progress and give and receive support. **Time - 10 minutes**

- Use apps like *Lift* to help you create and achieve new habits. **Time - 5 minutes**

Having a great morning routine is not just about making time for positive things, it's also about eliminating the negative things. They might not necessarily be bad things, but they are things that are best done once your day is already underway, rather than first thing in the morning. Each one of them can easily undo all your hard work and ruin your peace and calm.

Things to avoid in the morning

- **Morning news.** Most news is depressing, and it gives our day a negative and often emotional slant. ⬬ 11

- **Emails and other work-related things.** Checking in on work leaves you feeling overwhelmed from the get-go - not a great start.

- **Stimulants.** How many of us wake up with a cup of coffee, tea, or an energy drink in our hands? And yet it is actually counterproductive. Cortisol is one of the hormones that wakes us up, and first thing in the morning they are at their highest. The problem is, caffeine interferes with the production of cortisol, meaning we have to rely more and more on the caffeine.

  Unfortunately, drinking caffeine in the morning also means your body builds a tolerance to it, meaning it is less and less useful. So not only have you replaced cortisol with caffeine, that caffeine boost no longer works as well. Bummer, man.

  I adore tea. I blame my two years in England. But when I started getting headaches when I ran out of time for my morning cup, I realised that even that relatively small amount of caffeine wasn't doing me any favours. It is something I have now changed from a habit to an occasional enjoyment. It wasn't easy, but it was so worth it!

- **Sleeping in.** While sleeping in seemed like a big fat myth for a few years there, my daughter is now old enough that I can once again enjoy morning lie-ins on the weekend. Only problem? I end up feeling tired and sluggish for most of the morning. It's just not worth it.

Not only does it disrupt my morning routine, I find I have less motivation to get tasks done.

So now I compromise. I get up and do some work or exercise at 6, and when I come back I have a cup of tea in bed with my husband. This works far better. I still get to relax, but I have already achieved something and that has given me energy and a positive start to the day. Okay that's a big fat lie. I don't do this every weekend, but it's something I'm actively working on. I can definitely tell the difference between the days I lie in and those I don't though!

- **Social media and the Internet.** Not only do these two things consume huge amounts of valuable morning time, but like reading the news, they can start your day off negatively. Comparing your life to others instead of working towards your own goals is definitely not a great way to begin. Unless of course you have friends who post adorable fur baby pictures on Facebook. A little cuteness in the AM is always heart-warming.

A morning routine only needs to take 30 minutes. And it can change your whole day. I truly believe that making time for a good morning routine is one of the most important things you can do for your mood. The positivity it brings to your day far outweighs any other 'need' that you could use that time for. What else helps you achieve goals, relaxes your mind and body, helps you to connect with friends and family, lifts your self-esteem and self-worth, and creates a healthier body and mind?

* * *

RECAP ✄

- We should all have a morning routine. The average person is most productive when they first wake up, and how we start the day can set the pace and your emotional state for the rest of the day.

- A morning routine doesn't have to be hours long. Aim for just half an hour of uninterrupted time each day for great results.

- Setting a routine is one of the most powerful things you can do for your mood. Use the ideas listed in this chapter to create your own routine or include things that are important to you.

ACTION STEPS ✏

Do now:

- Write a list of everything you'd like to do in the mornings. You can use ideas from the list above or create your own.

- Create a morning routine for yourself using your list. Include the things that are the most important to you first, and don't overstretch yourself. It is better to continue doing a few things than to start with a huge amount and give up.

Plan to:

- Have an alarm that tells you when to go to sleep and when to wake. This is a simple way to get into a new habit.

- Switch yourself off at night - using the 'zero notifications method' so you are more alert in the mornings. ◎ 12

Work towards:

- Cutting out the things that negatively impact your morning.

- Adding in new morning routines as you create more time for yourself.

- Swapping out the things that don't work for those that do.

LINKED TO

1. A Positive Spin on Negative Thoughts

2. The Stressless S's

3. Eat the Food

4. Meditation is For Weirdos

5. Smile – Your Face Won't Crack

6. Say It Like You Mean It

7. Exercise Your Mind

8. Aim for the Stars

9. Give a Little

10. Social Butterfly

11. Unplug Your Brain

12. Successful Slumber

SUCCESSFUL SLUMBER
♪♫♪ IT'S A GREAT DAY TO BE ALIVE — TRAVIS TRITT ♪♫♪

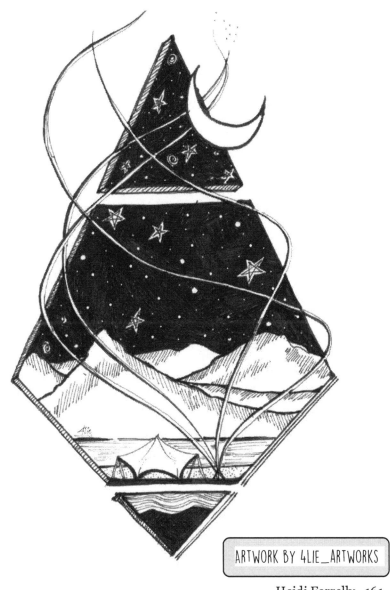

ARTWORK BY 4LIE_ARTWORKS

> *"Sleep is that golden chain that ties*
> *health and our bodies together."*
> -THOMAS DEKKER-

How amazing do you feel after a good night's sleep? Relaxed, rejuvenated, and ready to take on the world!

There's a reason for this. You haven't just wasted 8 hours of your life sleeping (although my husband would disagree) but have given your body and brain the only chance they get to do major repairs. You might be out for the count, but inside there is plenty going on. And if we deprive ourselves of this repair time it doesn't take long for sleep deprivation to start producing some pretty rubbish side effects.

Even one night of lost sleep can cause memory and concentration loss, severe yawning, poor moral judgment, impaired reaction time, and loss of coordination (kinda like being drunk only without the warm fuzzies). More than one night and our immune function also declines, and we have a higher risk of heart disease and obesity. Aches, tremors, and a risk of type 2 diabetes can also be bought on. We become irritable and lacking in energy. You can even start hallucinating!

Sleep deprivation is so bad it has been used as a form of torture since 1491, including the witch hunts of the 16th century, in the infamous gulags of Russia, and throughout the World Wars by various nations. Studies on sleep deprivation performed on puppies (seriously, people?!) found that lack of sleep was fatal. All the puppies died after 1-2 weeks of being kept awake.

And yet we don't prioritize sleep because it's not important? Man, have we got that wrong!

Even getting a couple of hours sleep less a night than you should can leave you with a massive 'sleep debt' that scientists are beginning to discover can have many of the same symptoms as sleep deprivation. And it can't just be made up with a lie in on the weekend either. 'All-nighters,' shift work, and insomnia, all have the same result. A steady decline in our body's health, our brains function, our mood, and our stress levels. So, nothing too serious...

> ☻ Sleep plays an important role in the brain, as the brain clears out waste by-products, balances neurotransmitters, and processes memories at rest. At both short and long extremes, rest may have an effect on mood and mental health.[20]

Sleep and stress have a two-way relationship. You know stress can interfere with your sleep, but did you know having a great sleep is one of the most important things you can do to reduce the effects of stress? Sleep is a fabulous way to eliminate stress from your body and refuel your brain. Think about how you feel after a good night's sleep. How about after a rough night?

Stress severely impacts our sleep, and many of us are not only highly stressed but not dealing with it on a day-to-day basis. Eliminating stress is vitally important for your health ⊘ 1 as stress perpetuates the vicious cycle of insomnia = stress, and stress = insomnia. Sleep allows the body's stress hormones to return to normal, so they're not depleted when we need them next, and gives us increased levels of patience to deal with life.

---

[20] http://www.huffingtonpost.com/rosie-osmun/oversleeping-the-effects-and-health-risks-of-sleeping-too-much_b_9092982.html

Small irritations and problems are much harder to cope with when you're tired, leading to (you guessed it), increased stress. So, **while working on diminishing stress is a great start to sleeping well, having a good bedtime routine is crucial to keeping those stress levels under wraps.** Exercise ◎ 2 and relaxation ◎ 3, while at opposite ends of the spectrum, are both incredibly important for eliminating stress and prioritizing your life can also help. ◎ 4

How many people do you know who consistently have great sleep? Knowing we need sleep and actually getting it are two very different things. Work, children, insomnia, sickness, lack of exercise, negative thinking, stress, they all interfere with our ability to get a great sleep. So, if you're one of the many people struggling with lack of sleep, here are a few tips to help you out.

- Establish a bedtime routine. A night-time routine is almost as important as a morning one. Your body loves routine. It loves knowing what it's doing when. And the better your routine, the quicker you will not only get to sleep, but enjoy a good night's sleep. Having a good night-time routine allows our minds to 'debrief' after a busy day, our bodies to relax, and our systems to reboot ready for a fresh start.

  Whether it's making lunches, folding washing, doing a crossword puzzle, or going for a gentle walk, find something you can do every night which will signal your body that it's almost sleep time. Slipping into a familiar routine before bed goes a long way towards helping get a great sleep.

- Keeping the same bedtime each night is also incredibly important. While doing the same things as a 'pre-bed winddown' each night is great, doing it at the same *time* each night is also vital. Your body loves the routine and rhythm of a set bedtime and goes into autopilot when you keep one. It knows when it should be producing melatonin, which helps you feel sleepy, and it's easier to fall asleep and stay asleep. Pick an hour you know you'll be able to stick to and set a couple of alarms to help you make it. A 'start your night time routine' alarm and a 'go to bed' alarm.

- If you need to eat or drink close to bedtime, try snacking on foods high in tryptophan, a sleep-promoting substance. Do you remember the old wives' tale of drinking a warm glass of milk before bed? Turns out it's pretty accurate. Dairy products are high in tryptophan, as are nuts, seeds, bananas, honey, and eggs. Carbs also increase the tryptophan in your blood. Keep your snack small though, or you'll be uncomfortable. A few crackers and cheese, or a spoonful of peanut butter maybe?

- Don't eat protein-heavy or high-fat meals like meat and takeaways just before bed. Not only is feeling full uncomfortable when you're trying to sleep, it can cause you to wake up in the night for bathroom breaks and disrupts sleep.

- Avoid all caffeine 4-6 hrs before bed. This includes tea, coffee, cola, and even hot chocolate. Some prescription medication can also contain caffeine, so make sure you check your labels.

- I love a nightcap as much as the next person, but unfortunately drinking alcohol before bed can give you nightmares, headaches, and a less restful sleep overall. Not to mention having to get up to use the bathroom. If you do drink, balance each glass of alcohol with a glass of water.

- Don't be fooled into thinking a quiet smoke before bed will calm you down, either. The nicotine in cigarettes is a stimulant just like caffeine and can have just as much impact on your sleep. If giving up is not on the agenda, then try to time your last cigarette for a couple of hours before bed.

- Don't watch a scary movie or listen to stimulating music before bed. Both of these are guaranteed to pep you up at a time you should be winding down.

- Don't make emotional calls at night. Not only is this guaranteed to put you on edge, but our judgment just isn't as good when we're tired, and you may end up wishing phones didn't exist by the time you get up in the morning. Not having that night cap should help with this... There's actually a few really cool apps that will lock your phone to certain numbers in case you have a willpower fail.

- While exercise is awesome, it's not great within a few hours of bed. It raises your temperature, your adrenaline levels, and your heart rate, none of which is great for feeling sleepy. The only exception are things like a gentle stroll or stretching that don't elevate your heart rate but relax you instead. Exercising earlier in the day, on the other hand, is great for sleep.

- Computers, phones, tablets, and even Kindles all emit what's known as blue light. Blue light interrupts our production of melatonin, the sleep-inducing hormone. Light suppresses melatonin, and interrupts our circadian rhythm, putting the whole body out of whack. 🔗5

Power down an hour before bed using the 'zero notifications method'. Switch off the TV, set phones and tablets to 'do not disturb' mode so you're not tempted to check those notifications, and read paper books instead of E-readers.

I use this hour before bed to pack work and school bags, make lunches, tidy the house, and wash dishes. (Sometimes. I hate doing dishes. They are my nemesis.) Doing odd jobs like these will provide you with that hour's 'down time' while still allowing you to get things done. Alternatively, you could play a board game with a family member, relax, craft, or simply chat. You might be surprised at how open your night becomes without screens right up 'til bedtime.

☢ A study done in 2014 showed that people reading on a tablet before bed instead of a printed book had more trouble getting to sleep, had less REM sleep (the phase when we dream), and were more alert before bed. They also had more trouble waking up, and were sleepier, even after the same length of sleep![21]

- It's not just blue light that's bad either. Even normal household lighting can disrupt your body's melatonin production. I mean, clearly if it's bright it's still daytime, right? No need to start producing sleepy hormones. If possible, keep your lights to a minimum an hour before bed. Soft lamps and candles work well. Many candle scents like lavender are also great for relieving stress too, so you'll kill two birds with one stone.

---

[21] http://www.pnas.org/content/112/4/1232

- Don't fall asleep on the sofa! Or anywhere else except your bed. Remember, you're trying to build good sleep habits, and you want your body to know that bed is the place to nod off. If you find yourself getting drowsy, then head to your room. It doesn't matter if it's 'too early.' Your body knows what it needs, and what's the difference between sleeping on the lounge at 8 or sleeping in bed?

- On the other end of the spectrum... Don't get into bed until you're feeling drowsy. It's all very well having a routine, but spending an extra 15 minutes winding down could help you fall asleep faster than if you get into bed earlier but wide awake.

- Calm your mind before bed. There is absolutely no point trying to get to sleep if you're wired from a busy day. If you exercise late, are still tucking kids into bed at 9 p.m., or working up until bedtime, then chances are while your body is exhausted, your brain is zinging! How many of us go to bed at night tuckered out, only to lie awake unable to drift off?

  Try reading magazines or simple non-fiction books like cookbooks until you get drowsy (not fiction books, or you'll get sucked into a plot line). Do a crossword or puzzle, try some adult colouring, or do some sleep yoga (yes, there is such a thing).

  Do all of this in your lounge room or another quiet spot that isn't your bedroom. Use your bedroom for sleep (and sex) only. Don't read in bed, chat on the phone, bring work into your bedroom, or hide there looking for a quiet moment on Facebook. We want to program our minds into a bed = sleep mentality, so that we fall asleep faster, stay asleep longer, and have a better night's sleep overall. Sounds amazing, right?

- If you get into bed and find yourself lying awake for 15 minutes or more, get up. You're not doing yourself any favours, and the longer you lie there tossing and turning, the less your brain associates bed with sleep, and the more it links it to frustration.

  I often leave a basket of clean washing in the lounge to fold. (I don't know how we go through so much washing. There's only 3 of us, for goodness' sake!) This way if I can't sleep I get up, fold washing till I feel drowsy, and then head back to bed, and 9 times out of 10 this will work and I will drop off. Of course, when I go straight to sleep every night it means I have to fold the washing during the day like every other person. Sigh.

  Reading, folding washing, or anything else you're doing when you'd normally be in bed, all cuts into that precious sleep time. But not only are you likely to get more sleep by getting up, you build much better sleep habits long-term than by lying in bed awake. And nothing makes your mood plummet more than watching the clock tick ever onwards without being able to sleep! On that note, get rid of your clock if you can, or put it somewhere you can't see it.

- Do you fall asleep fast, only to wake in the wee hours with your mind racing? Have headphones ready next to your bed, so you can listen to some calming music, white noise, or play a meditation app. Try tapping as a way to turn off negative or chaotic thoughts ✪ 6 and move your focus elsewhere, or wake your partner for a shag (they're not usually disgruntled). If you do need to get up, keep lights off or to a minimum and don't do anything that will make you too alert.

- Write down your worries before bed. This way they will not be floating around in your head all night. Once you have them on paper, come up with 3 things you could do to either combat the issue or see it from a different angle. Once you've done that, tear/burn/otherwise destroy your list of troubles. This is a proven technique for showing your brain that they are not important. If you're prone to rumination⊘7 then make sure you have an affirmation⊘8 ready to stop your brain continuing its vicious cycle.

- The same is true for grand ideas. Write them down. If you're like me and have epiphanies just as you're falling asleep then keep a pen and pad beside your bed. I've learnt that I fall asleep faster if I jot them down. You don't even have to turn the light on, just jot a quick note and snuggle back into bed. This way your thoughts stop churning, and you have a higher chance of nodding off.

- Journal the day's good moments, both big and small. Don't write a single bad thing about your day even if you think it was terrible! It doesn't matter how small, or how hard you have to look to find something, write only the good. This will help you focus your mind on the good in your day, instead of reinforcing the bad by writing them down. You can then look back at previous days and see your collection of happy memories. ⊘9

- Make sure you're getting plenty of B vitamins in your diet.⊘10 Vitamin B-6 helps convert some of the tryptophan in your body to vitamin B-3, and serotonin, both of which help regulate your sleep patterns. A deficiency in B-6 can cause insomnia and disturbed sleep patterns, as it disrupts your body's metabolism of the tryptophan, so getting enough is incredibly important.

- If you're still struggling to sleep, take a look at magnesium. According to research, "Magnesium plays an important role in hydration, muscle relaxation, energy production and, crucially, the deactivation of adrenaline." And most of us are deficient in magnesium. Did you know it takes 54 magnesium molecules to get rid of just one sugar molecule? No wonder we're all so deficient! Natural Calm, and other products like it, can help people sleep where many other things have failed. Give it a try. It's a simple and tasty solution. My daughter's always trying to steal mine!

- A popular sleep aid that can be taken in the form of tea is an herbal sedative called passionflower. While clinical trials in humans are lacking, what experiments have been done have shown enhanced sleep quality in participants.[22] It's also proven to be beneficial for reducing symptoms of insomnia, anxiety, and depression in menopausal women.[23] So if this is you, then consider a daily cup of passionflower tea!

Sleeping pills

If you've ever taken them, you know they can be a godsend for sleepless nights. But you'll also know they can leave you feeling drowsy, achy, and come with a whole host of less than awesome side effects. Sleeping pills are also highly addictive, and while they are a 'quick fix,' they can act erratically in your brain. Sleep scientist and neurologist at Harvard Medical School,

---

[22] https://www.ncbi.nlm.nih.gov/pubmed/21294203
[23] https://www.ncbi.nlm.nih.gov/pubmed/22049281

Patrick Fuller, believes most people who take sleeping pills would actually have better results by using the techniques we talk about in this chapter.

> ☢ "They're not this cute little thing that comes in and targets a little cell in your brain that's just all involved in sleep. These drugs are not that specific; they affect not just the brain, but the peripheral systems as well. Sleeping pills are also highly addictive and getting off of them is tough because your insomnia or other sleeping problems may actually become worse after taking them. For the average Joe who's having a little trouble sleeping, there's a lot of things they can try to do to facilitate normal, natural sleep before popping Z-class drugs [common insomnia medications] at night." [24]

If you feel you have to use sleeping pills, do so with caution, and work towards weaning yourself off them by using sleep techniques instead.

Melatonin

Melatonin is a supplement taken by many people to help them sleep. It is produced by the body, so it's often viewed as safer than sleeping tablets - and that's what it's been marketed as. The 'all-natural sleep aid.'

However, **not only is melatonin a hormone that you are haphazardly putting into your system, there is actually no proof it helps with insomnia.** That's not what its purpose is.

---

[24] http://www.businessinsider.com/sleeping-pills-sleep-aid-safety-2016-2/?r=AU&IR=T

Melatonin is a sleep and body clock regulator – NOT a sleep initiator. Melatonin works with your biological clock by telling your brain when it is time to sleep. Melatonin does not increase your sleep drive or need for sleep.

– MICHAEL BREUS -

☢ Dr Richard Wurtman (the MIT neuroscientist who patented melatonin 21 years ago) has this to say about it. "Our bodies naturally produce "endogenous" melatonin (or, "growing or originating from within an organism")." What ends up on pharmacy shelves is synthesized "exogenous" melatonin — growing or originating from *outside* an organism. Melatonin supplements may work at first, but soon "you'll stop responding because you desensitize the brain. And as a consequence, not only won't you respond to the stuff you take... you won't respond to the stuff you make, so it can actually promote insomnia after a period of time." [25]

I found out firsthand the knock-on effect taking melatonin has several years ago when I was plagued with insomnia. I would go to sleep just fine but wake up at 2 or 3 in the morning and be wide awake. I started taking melatonin and it made me sleepier at night but didn't stop me from waking up. And then I started to have trouble even falling asleep... The bottom line is, it is better to use diet and lifestyle changes first and keep hormone replacement as a last resort.

---

[25] https://vanwinkles.com/the-dark-side-downsides-side-effects-of-melatonin

No chapter on sleep would be complete if we didn't talk about oversleeping. It seems like a dream to most - sleeping too much. But the health ramifications for oversleeping can be just as bad as those for not sleeping enough! Depression, anxiety, pain, inflammation, and degenerative diseases, to name just a few. It can even make you tireder! If you're struggling with oversleeping, try some of the following:

- Wake up to sunshine

- Avoid napping throughout the day

- Set up a good morning routine that begins early. This will help motivate you. ⊘ 11

- Get to bed by 10 p.m. as the 90-minute sleep phase before midnight is one of the most refreshing, leaving you feeling better rested in the morning.

- Make sure your body isn't trying to tell you about something else that's wrong, physically or emotionally.

- Eat breakfast within 30 minutes of rising. It increases your metabolism and promotes better sleep at night.

- Get more exercise.

- Put your alarm clock somewhere where you have to get up to turn it off. This means you can't just keep hitting snooze!

Like all routines, consistency is the key to making them work. Having a routine that you only follow one day a week is not going to help. Your body needs around 2 months for new routines to become habits ⊘ 12, so make sure the things you implement are sustainable. Sleep is essential to our well-being, and getting a good night's sleep, every night, is one of the most important things you can do for your mood. Start prioritizing it in your life!

It's pretty flippin' difficult to be happy and positive when you're cranky and struggling to stay awake. I cannot stress how important sleep is to your brain, your body, and your life.

Seriously people, sleep!

* * *

RECAP 📌

- Sleep gives your body and brain the only chance they get to do major repairs. Even one night of lost sleep can cause memory and concentration loss, poor judgement, impaired reaction time and loss of coordination. Sleep deprivation is so bad it has been used as a form of torture since 1491!

- Sleep is a fabulous way to eliminate stress from your body and refuel your brain. It allows your stress hormones to return to normal so they're not depleted when you need them next.

- Keeping the same bedtime each night is incredibly important. Find something you can do every night which will signal your body that it's almost sleep time and don't mess it up by falling asleep on the sofa!

- Avoiding caffeine 4-6 hrs before bed, snacking on foods high in tryptophan, writing down your worries and ideas and powering down an hour before bed all help you sleep better.

- Sleeping pills are highly addictive and can act erratically in your brain. And most people who take them would actually have better results by using the techniques we talk about in this chapter.

- The health ramifications for oversleeping can be just as bad as those for not sleeping enough!

ACTION STEPS ✎

Do now:

- Set a specific time that you can aim to be in bed every night. Make sure it is sustainable for your life, and not just built on ideals.

- Write a list of things you could do in the hour before bed instead of looking at screens.

- Write a list of quiet activities you could do if you need to get out of bed in the night.

- Make sure you are familiar with tapping and affirmations so you can use them to focus and calm your mind.

Plan to:

- Have a meditation app, simple activities, or quiet music ready if you wake up in the wee hours and need to switch off your mind.

- Use candles or lamps around the house at bedtime instead of bright lights.

- Minimise stimulants in your diet several hours before bed.

- Identify things in your environment that interfere with your sleep and start minimizing them.

Work towards:

- Following your sleep routine nightly until it becomes ingrained.

- Getting your optimal amount of sleep - usually somewhere between 7-9 hours. Not too much, not too little.

LINKED TO

1. The Stressless S's

2. Exercise Your Mind

3. Relaxation is a Real Thing

4. Sort Your Crazy

5. Unplug Your Brain

6. The Weird and The Wonderful

7. Thinking too Much About Crap You Shouldn't

8. Say it Like you Mean It

9. Great Attitude

10. Eat the Food

11. Get Out of Bed You Daisy Head

12. Routinely Amazing

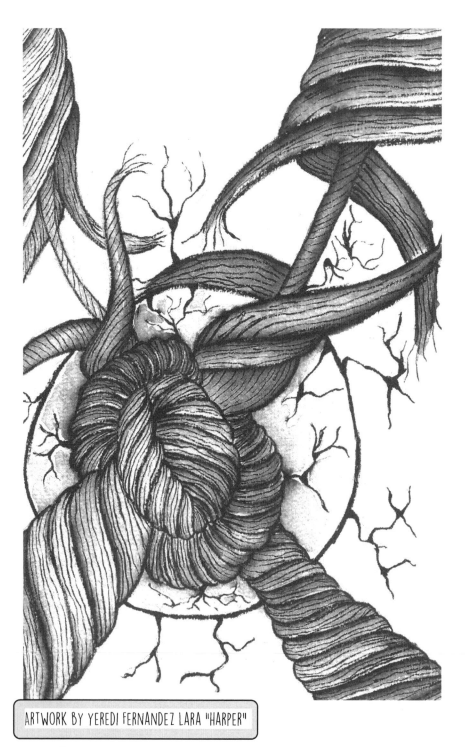

ARTWORK BY YEREDI FERNANDEZ LARA "HARPER"

STRESS

STRESS IS ONE OF THE BIGGEST CONTRIBUTING FACTORS TO LOW MOOD. LIKE A CANCER, IT SEEMS TO INVADE EVERY AREA OF YOUR LIFE AND TWINES ITSELF SO TIGHTLY THAT IT JUST BECOMES 'NORMAL'. OUR SEDENTARY, BUSY, UNHEALTHY LIFESTYLES CREATE A CYCLE OF STRESS THAT IS NOT ONLY DAMAGING BUT SELF—PERPETUATING.

BUT THERE **ARE** WAYS TO COMBAT STRESS IF YOU KNOW HOW!

THE STRESSLESS S'S
♪♫♪ GOOD FEELING – FLO RIDA ♪♫♪

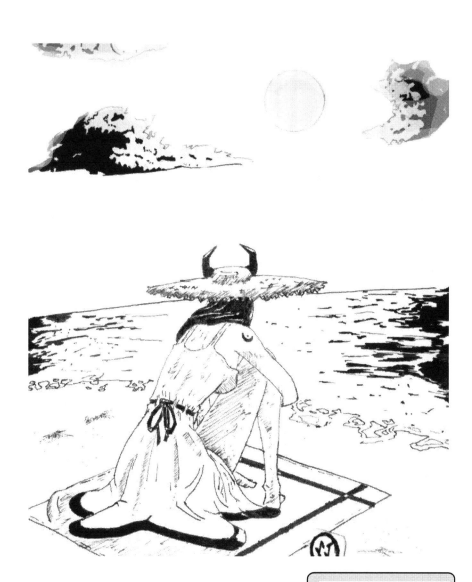

ARTWORK BY JOSE JAIMES

What do sunlight, sea water, and sex all have in common? Well, other than starting with S, they are all incredible stress relievers and mood boosters.

Stress is one of the biggest contributing factors for low mood, and in today's crazy world we are being exposed to more of it than ever before. Stress is the body's reaction to particular situations such as:

- The death of a loved one

- Moving house

- Getting married

- Traveling

- Financial problems

- Relationship issues

- Fear and panic

- Emotional issues such as depression

- Unrealistic expectations of yourself and others

- Focusing on the negative

- Retirement

- Injury or illness

Stress is not always bad. It is your body's way of responding to danger or the demands that are placed on it. It is the classic fight-or-flight reaction, and short term it can help us through difficult situations and challenges. When stress sticks around though, it can become an issue.

Stress creates adrenaline and histamine, both of which have a big impact on the body. Adrenaline can only be expelled from the body through hard physical exercise, yet many highly stressed people are also highly sedentary. The stressed mind then starts to manifest itself as illnesses of the body.

Whether your stress is generated from work, life, or yourself, is irrelevant. Your body doesn't differentiate, and it still has to process it. And this can lead to all sorts of health problems such as insomnia, heart disease, depression, weight problems, autoimmune diseases, and pain.

☢ The fight-or-flight stress response is the body's answer to perceived threat or danger. During this reaction, certain hormones like adrenalin and cortisol are released, speeding the heart rate, slowing digestion, shunting blood flow to major muscle groups, and changing various other autonomic nervous functions, giving the body a burst of energy and strength. Originally named for its ability to enable us to physically fight or run away when faced with danger, it's now activated in situations where neither response is appropriate, like in traffic or during a stressful day at work. When the perceived threat is gone, systems are designed to return to normal function via the relaxation response, but in our times of chronic stress, this often doesn't happen enough, causing damage to the body. [26]

There are many things you can do to help combat stress in your life. We discuss many of them in other chapters of *Choosing Happy*. Relaxation, Exercise, Goal Setting, Routines, Food, Socialization, Spirituality, Sleep, Switching Off, Meditation, and Gratitude ⌗ 1 all help diminish stress before it gets a stranglehold. But there are other things that can help too.

SUN

Sunlight is one of my favourites! If there is such a thing as a past life I think I would have been a cat or a lizard. I love the sun! I love relaxing in a sunny spot and am always happier on

---

[26] http://www.youngdiggers.com.au/fight-or-flight

sunny days. Which is not surprising. Studies have proven exposure to sunlight can significantly brighten your mood, and lack of it can make you feel sluggish, moody, and downright depressed.

So, what's the answer? Get into the sun more! Vitamin D (which is produced when sunlight has access to your skin) is vital for stimulating serotonin. Serotonin in turn regulates mood, appetite, sleep, and memory. It adjusts your body clock for optimal function and regulates circadian rhythms.

People who suffer from SAD (seasonal affective disorder) are particularly affected by lack of light and sunshine during the winter months. And studies have shown that these people, when exposed to light, especially in the morning, tend to feel better! [27]

> ☻ "The farther north from the equator you live, the greater the risk you'll have some degree of winter depression. 'SAD' - or 'seasonal depression' as it's been coined, is felt by only about 1.5% of Florida residents, compared to about 10% of those living in New Hampshire."[28]

Many of us have become so worried about the sun that when we are outdoors we are covered from head to toe. Which is fabulous in Australia in the middle of the summer, but not necessary in the early morning, late afternoon, or in the winter. Yes, continue safe sun practices, but also **remember that sunshine is incredibly important to our health and get out in it whenever it's safe to do so.**

---

[27] http://www.huffingtonpost.com.au/entry/climate-health_n_4568505
[28] www.normanrosenthal.com/seasomal-affective-disorder/

Some countries like New Zealand have a UV index, which alerts you when the ultraviolet rays from the sun are at 3 or above. Use this as a gauge for when you need sun protection and when you don't. Otherwise, the general rule of thumb is that the sun is at its harshest after 10 a.m. and before 3 p.m. Here's some tips for getting into the sun more:

- If you work in an office, or somewhere where you don't see or feel the sunshine, then make sure you get out in it during your breaks.

- Have your lunch in natural sunlight.

- Get off the bus early and walk in the sun.

- Have your breakfast on your balcony or front lawn.

- Go for a walk first thing in the morning or in late afternoon.

- Open drapes and windows and let the sunshine in!

- Practice safe sunbathing. You shouldn't even feel a bite from the sun, let alone get burnt. It is simply allowing the sun onto your skin when it is at its mildest.

- Learn to live without sunglasses. This is something I really struggle with. I live in Australia and my sunnies are on my face or on top of my head all day. I can now do without them morning and afternoon, and I definitely sleep better when I don't wear them. (See the science box for more info).

- If you can't get into the sun during the working week then make sure you have less screen time and more green time on the weekends.

☢ When full-spectrum light enters your eyes, it not only goes to your visual centres enabling you to see, it also goes to your brain's hypothalamus where it impacts your entire body. Your hypothalamus controls body temperature, hunger and thirst, water balance, and blood pressure. Additionally, it controls your body's master gland, the pituitary, which secretes many essential hormones, including those that influence your mood. Exposure to full-spectrum lighting is actually one effective therapy used for treating depression, infection, and much more. [29]

Your hypothalamus is also connected to the pineal gland. The pineal gland is largely responsible for regulating your sleep/wake cycles via the secretion of melatonin (the good sleep hormone). The natural contrast of light during the day and night that your body (and eyes) are exposed to helps assure healthy hormonal secretions and healthy sleep. Sunglasses inhibit this process. It's a simple as that. [30]

SEA & SALT

My husband once said to me that surfing is one of the only sports people can watch for hours, even if they're not really interested in it. Why? The ocean. Just being around the sea and hearing the waves crash onto the shore is relaxing, and awe inspiring. And when we swim in the ocean, or in sea pools (man-made pools the ocean fills at high tide), we not only get that calmness, but physical attributes as well.

- Sea water helps heal sores, eczema, and acne.

---

[29]
https://articles.mercola.com/sites/articles/archive/2013/09/16/sunglasses-myths.aspx
[30] http://theshawnstevensonmodel.com/side-effects-of-sunglasses/

- Swimming in the ocean improves our circulatory system, bringing more oxygen to the brain, to make us more alert and active.

- Gargling salt water helps with sore throats.

- The sound of waves alters wave patterns in the brain, lulling you into a deeply relaxed state to rejuvenate the mind and body. This is why many people use the sound of ocean waves to sleep by.

- Salt water opens the pores and allows sea minerals to be absorbed, and toxins to be expelled.

- Minerals such as potassium and magnesium are restored by swimming in sea water, and help balance calcium, calm the nervous system, and relieve stress.

If you don't live near the ocean, hunt around for an indoor pool that uses salt instead of chlorine. It's not quite as good, but still much better than nothing! Drinking a glass of water with a little added rock or sea salt is also an option. This little trick also helps eliminate fatigue, stabilize blood pressure, and reduce appetite. Go easy on it though - it is also a diuretic!

Salt has long been known for its restorative properties and is not necessarily the villain it is portrayed to be. Most of the salt present in processed food is table salt - villainize that all you want, it's definitely as bad as it's made out. But rock and sea salt are very good for many areas of your body, and most of us just aren't getting enough of it in our diets anymore.

Swimming in general is also great for your body as it is easy on your joints, reduces inflammation, and helps with aches and pains. But when you swim in the ocean you combine all these benefits with those from fresh air and sunshine, and the minerals and salt the ocean contains. Perfect.

SEX

Physical and emotional connection is critical for almost all of us 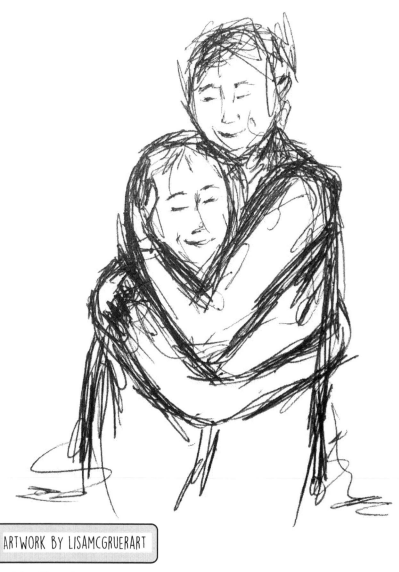 2, and sex is about as connected as you can get! Sex boosts both physical and mental health (as long as you're practicing safe sex - there's no excuse not to these days), and regular sex (1-2 times a week), helps reduce stress, boost self-esteem, and increases the bond with your partner.

ARTWORK BY LISAMCGRUERART

I'm not suggesting you run out and start hooking up with random people, this is about as detrimental to your health as you can get! But if you're already in a relationship, then stop looking for excuses not to shag, and make it happen!

Stress can really dampen your libido, and leave you wanting sex less and less. Which is annoying because sex helps boost libido! If you need to, start with some of the other stress relievers, and you'll soon be looking forward to sex more. And remember, the more you do it, the more you'll want to, so make an effort even if you're not enthralled by the idea.

If the thought of sex with your partner really revolts you, you never seem to have free time together (you need to work on this, man!), or you're single, think about self-pleasure. ▶ While it doesn't give you the physical connection that having sex with a partner does, it is still a great way to relieve stress, and teaches you to love yourself and your body.

Sex also has a range of other benefits:

- Sex helps boost your heart rate, improve your flexibility, and burn calories as it is similar to moderate exercise.

- Regular sex is great for your heart health and can help fight heart disease.

- Regular sex also improves your body's immune system.

- Sexual activity releases pain-reducing hormones that can help diminish all types of pain including headaches. That headache is really not an excuse now...

- Sex helps build women's pelvic floor muscles, which is great news if you've had kids, or have trouble with incontinence.

- Sex is linked to better stress response and lower blood pressure.

- 2 types of hormones released during orgasm (not just sex – orgasm, people), promote sleep and help you nod off more quickly. So, don't be so hard on your partner when he's snoring soon after. It's what your body was designed to do!

Sex is not only great for a healthy mind and body, but for that all important physical and emotional connection. Get into it!

* * *

RECAP ✎

- Stress is one of the biggest contributing factors for low mood. It's your body's reaction to particular situations such as the death of a loved one, financial problems, or fear and panic.

- Stress is not always bad. Short term it can help us through difficult situations and challenges. But when we are constantly stressed our body never has a chance to return to normal function.

- Sunshine is incredibly important to your health and an excellent stress reliever. Exposure to sunlight can significantly brighten your mood, and lack of it can make you feel sluggish, moody, and downright depressed. If you can't get into the sun during the working week then make sure you have less screen time and more green time on the weekends.

- Salt has long been known for its restorative properties, and getting salt from the ocean is twice as effective because just being around the sea and hearing the waves crash onto the shore is relaxing. When you swim in salt water minerals such as potassium and magnesium are restored, and it also helps balance calcium, the nervous system, and relieve stress.

- Sex is not only great for a healthy body and mind but for that all important physical and emotional connection. Regular sex helps reduce stress, boost self-esteem and libido, and increases the bond with your partner.

ACTION STEPS ✎

Do now:

- Make a list of all the ways you can get more sunshine in your life. If possible, combine them with other things such as exercise, sea swimming, socializing, or learning a new skill.

- If it's daytime go outside and get some sun. Not under layers of clothing, glasses, and sunscreen, but old school, on your skin. Crazy! (Be sensible and remember the sun should never even bite, let alone burn.)

- Work out how you can get more salt into your life. Preferably through ocean swimming, but anything is better than nothing!

- If you're at home with your partner, drag them off for a quick shag. If you're not, wait until you have a free moment and seize it!!

Plan to:

- Spend time in the sun. Early morning sun is the best for mood. Face the sun between 7 a.m. and 10 a.m. without sunscreen, clothing, or sunglasses getting in the way. If it's too bright close your eyes, the sunshine still gets in. Be sensible and only sit in the sun when you know you're not going to burn, and only for 10-15 minutes, 2-3 times a week.

- Introduce ocean swimming into your life and start using sea salt in your diet.

- Make more of an effort when it comes to sex. Not only will your body and mind be healthier, your relationship with your partner and yourself will be too.

Work towards:

- Having time in the sun every day.

- Swimming in the ocean or a salt pool once a week. Or at the very least, getting more salt in your diet. The good stuff, not that nasty table salt.

- Having safe, *orgasmic* sex with a trusted partner twice a week.

LINKED TO

1. Relaxation is a Real Thing
   Exercise Your Mind
   Aim for the Stars
   Routinely Amazing
   Eat the Food!
   Social Butterfly
   Spiritual Value
   Successful Slumber
   Unplug Your Brain
   Meditation is for Weirdos
   Great Attitude

2. Social Butterfly

RELAXATION IS A REAL THING
♪♫♪ BEAUTIFUL DAY – U2 ♪♫♪

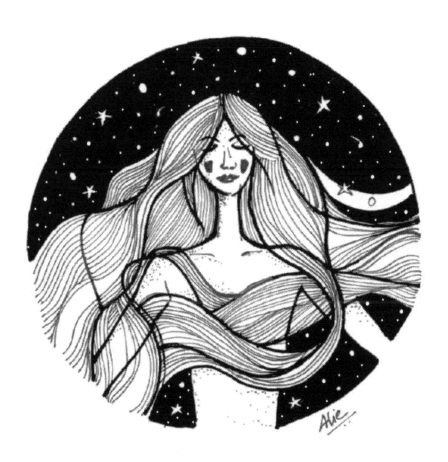

ARTWORK BY 4LIE_ARTWORKS

I am a 'typical' woman in that I love to relax and have some quiet time. Pampering is even better. But it almost never happens. Why? Because I don't make time for it. I work part time, I run a house, I work from home, and I am always putting other things first. I'm not being a martyr, it's just the way it is. It is the same reason I didn't exercise regularly for years after the birth of my daughter.

Except it's not a reason. Not really. It's an excuse. **Relaxation is vital to our health and wellbeing and yet it is an almost forgotten art.**

Women are their own worst enemies. The majority of us are too busy, so we get stressed, and yet we're not making time for the things that can really help relieve that stress because we're too busy. Exercise, relaxation, and personal time, to name just a few. Cycle of stress, anyone?

When we do chisel out some relaxation time, we feel rushed, or guilty for doing something for ourselves. Sometimes I think we feel if we just get enough work, chores, meals, etc., done today, we'll have free time to relax and exercise tomorrow. But that's never the case!

There will always be work to do, no matter what form it takes. And the only thing we're doing by putting ourselves last is screwing up our minds and bodies. This causes us to be stressed, unhappy, and worn out, which in turn means we don't get as much done. See what I'm saying? Not looking after yourself, not exercising, and not putting yourself first - it's counterproductive!

We need to prioritize ourselves. We are incredibly important. The people around us may need us, and rely on us, but that only makes it more important to look after ourselves first.

One of the hardest things for me to learn when I became a mum was making time for myself. There was always so much to do that I was constantly overwhelmed and never had a quiet moment. And this is not limited to mums. I know plenty of working men and women who spend all week at work and then all weekend working around the home. Not only is this unhealthy, it is unsustainable, and a recipe for low mood. Life is not exactly fun when the only thing you ever do is work, and stress about the work you haven't done!

☢ Downtime replenishes the brain's stores of attention and motivation, encourages productivity and creativity, and is essential to both achieve our highest levels of performance and simply form stable memories in everyday life. A wandering mind unsticks us in time so that we can learn from the past and plan for the future. Moments of respite may even be necessary to keep one's moral compass in working order and maintain a sense of self.[31]

When I was going through a bad patch I had this one conversation with my husband that I will never forget. He was trying to tell me to get out more, to see friends, do exercise, and enjoy life. That my happiness was in my hands and I had the power to change it. I told him through my (seemingly ever present) tears that I didn't have time, after doing the washing, cooking, cleaning, and day-to-day chores.

He gave me this incredulous look and said, "Stop doing them! I don't care if I come home and the house is a mess and we have to heat pies for dinner, as long as you've had a nice day and are happy." Yup. He's pretty amazing. Not everyone has such a

---

[31] https://www.scientificamerican.com/article/mental-downtime/

supportive spouse, and even those that do will probably find the same thing I did. They have to get past their guilt first.

You see, my husband works full time, and he works hard. Then he comes home and often does work around the house. I also work, but only part time. I have 3 days a week where I do all the chores, do the school and activity runs, and write. Technically, I can spend this time seeing friends, catching a movie, or going for a swim at the beach. But I never did! Because even though my days are full, and my evenings and weekends often are too, I felt so guilty that I was enjoying the sun when he was at work that I just didn't do it.

The upshot of that, of course, was that I ended up being busy all the time, and never doing anything for myself. In the weekends, we went to the beach so my husband could surf because he had been at work all week, and I still did the day-to-day chores. It took my husband pointing out this (seemingly obvious) fact for me to see it. Just because I don't go to work 5 days a week doesn't mean I don't work as hard. Who cares if the house is spotless and yesterday's clothes are washed if you are miserable?

Clearly, I'm a bit slow on the uptake, but I finally realised that if I wanted to enjoy my life, then I had to let go of guilt ⊘ 1. I learnt to prioritize my life by what was important rather than what was expected. And if spending a couple of hours by myself on those 3 days I had free of work and children gave me my own time back, as well as my sanity, then that was time well spent.

"Time you enjoy wasting, is not wasted."
MARTHE TROLY-CURTIN

Letting go of guilt didn't happen overnight. I still have days where I come home covered in sand from the beach, and my husband comes home covered in grease, and my brain tells me I'm a horrible person. But I'm learning to ignore that annoying little voice because I know my husband is right. I do work hard. And enjoying myself in no way makes me less of a person. It simply makes me human, and happy. And that is what life is all about.

This doesn't mean you have a free pass to be lazy. And it certainly doesn't mean that someone else should be working harder because you're working less. It just means that instead of always putting everything and everyone else first, you put yourself first on a regular basis. You let go of the things that don't really matter, and you prioritize your life so that happiness comes before work. Check out the "Jar of Life" analogy in Sort Your Crazy ✪ 2, for a great example.

Look at it this way. When you're sitting on a plane listening to the safety demonstration and they tell you, "When oxygen masks fall from the ceiling, please put on your own mask before you try to help anyone else," what do you think? Do you immediately think, "That's ridiculous. I'll put other people's on first?" No! Of course not. Because you know you can't help anyone if you've passed out from lack of oxygen.

This is what I mean by putting yourself first. **You are better able to help and be of service to others if you look after yourself first.** So, you need to ask yourself, not just today, but every day: Have I looked after myself yet today?

But what if you work full time, and you're trying to be a good parent? Or if you hold down 3 jobs just to make ends meet? What then? Surely relaxation isn't as important as putting food on the table! It is. Because if you never, ever relax then at some point you are going to get sick or fall apart. And all those little balls you're juggling in the air are going to come crashing down.

Relaxation doesn't need to be a whole day affair. It could be just getting up 10 minutes earlier and having a cup of tea while watching the sun rise. There are so many things we can do on a daily basis that will relax and de-stress us. And you only need 10-30 minutes for most of them. There is no valid reason for not making time on a regular basis for yourself. See Sort Your Crazy and Routinely Awesome @ 3 for ways to make this happen. Without interruption!

Here's some things many people find relaxing. Use this list to prompt your memory and help you rediscover what you love.

- Walking in nature or enjoying your local countryside

- Listening to the ocean, or walking on the beach

- Gardening

- Sitting in the morning sun @ 4

- Reading a simple book, magazine, or newspaper

- Having a quiet cuppa

- Dancing

- Singing or listening to music @ 5 (pick carefully)

- Meditating @ 6

- Spending time with good friends and family @ 7

- Watching a movie/TV show

- Eating good meals

- Thinking about something good that will happen in the future

- Do a simple crossword

- Do some knitting, cross-stitch, or sewing

- Listen to something funny or interesting on the radio or a podcast

- Find a new recipe to try

- Stroke or groom your pet

- Wash and style your hair

- Manicure your nails

- Draw or paint

- Soak your feet and do a pedicure

- Play a game or do a puzzle

- Take some photographs

Not only does making time for yourself have a positive effect on you, but on those around you. Science suggests that caring about our own happiness isn't merely selfish or indulgent, it seems to be contagious. If we're relaxed and happy, those around us are more likely to be happy, and we tend to help others more. [32]

Sometimes, small moments are not enough though. If you find yourself fidgeting when you're relaxing, if your mind wanders when you're trying to read, if you're still thinking of jobs when you're at a café, then you're not actually relaxing. You're just going through the motions.

If this is you, then you need to take a good hard look at your life. Why aren't you happy? What is causing you the most stress? Taking up the most time? What do you need to change in your life to make those moments of relaxation work for you? Perhaps small changes aren't enough. Maybe you need to look at making a big change.

---

[32] https://hms.harvard.edu/news/harvard-medicine/contagion-happiness

Making large changes in our lives can be terrifying. But they can also bring freedom, exhilaration, and a newfound love for life. If you are miserable in your job, your relationship, or the direction your life is heading, then change it! It's not just going to miraculously right itself. You have to take steps to ensure it does.

"Twenty years from now you will be more disappointed by the things that you didn't do than by the ones you did. So, throw off the bowlines. Sail away from safe harbour. Catch the trade winds in your sails. Explore. Dream. Discover."
– MARK TWAIN -

Sometimes making big changes means sacrificing other things. My husband gave up a secure job he hated, and which made him miserable, to work as a contractor. He doesn't have the same job security, but he is so much happier, and looking back now, we would still make the same decision again.

Our bid to pay off our mortgage in 10 years has meant giving up a lot of things people take for granted. Eating out, new clothes, holidays abroad. These are all things we have put on the back burner, not because we didn't want them, but because prioritizing our mortgage was more important to our future happiness. This was how we chose to alter our lives for the better.

Perhaps you will have to spend time on minimum wage while you retrain, or simply have a break from your chosen profession. Perhaps you will be lonely, or scared, or uncertain about your future. But holding a course just because it is known, or safe, doesn't bring you happiness. Sometimes you need to make big changes in your life, so you can remember and enjoy the little things you love and find relaxing

In the end, it is up to us to make relaxation a priority. And if this means you need to make changes (big or small) to learn how to relax, then do it! Even if it's only one small step at a time.

* * *

RECAP 📌

- Not looking after yourself, not exercising, and not putting yourself first on a daily basis is counterproductive. Relaxation is vital to our health and wellbeing.

- You are better able to help and be of service to others if you look after yourself first. Who cares if the house is spotless and your 'to do' list is completed if you are miserable? Relaxation doesn't mean having a free pass to be lazy. It simply means you value yourself enough to look after your mind and body.

- Relaxation doesn't need to be a whole day affair. You might take 10 minutes to have a cup of tea and watch the sun rise. You might go for a swim at the beach or have a run in your lunch break. You might organise drinks with friends you haven't seen for a while. You only need 10-30 mins a day to relax and de-stress.

- Sometimes you need to make large changes in your life before you can truly relax.

- Making time for yourself has a positive effect on everyone. If we are relaxed and happy, those around us are more likely to be happy too.

- There is no valid reason for not making time on a regular basis for yourself.

ACTION STEPS ✎

Do now:

- Make a list of all the things that make you feel happy, relaxed, or give you a sense of achievement, even if it's only for a moment. Use the chapters in this book, and the list above to help you. You can categorize your list into body, mind, spirit if you like.

- Do one thing right now that makes you happy. It could be having an uninterrupted shower, a hot cup of tea, or going for a walk. Do it!

Plan to:

- Do at least one of the things in each category of your list every day.

- Keep a notepad next to your bed and write down everything you think of that helped you relax or de-stress that day. The things, people, and activities that made you just that little bit happier and calmer. Then start working them into your daily routine.

- Ask yourself each week: Am I looking after myself, my soul, my health, the very state of my being? When is the last time I did something purely for myself? If you haven't been prioritizing yourself, then start!

Work towards:

- Doing one thing every day for no other reason than you enjoy it.

- Finding a balance between other people's needs, work, and yourself.

LINKED TO 🔗

1. Emotional Rollercoaster

2. Sort Your Crazy

3. Routinely Amazing

4. The Stressless S's

5. Create a Song and Dance

6. Meditation is for Weirdos

7. Social Butterfly

MEDITATION IS FOR WEIRDOS

♪♫♪ I GOTTA FEELING — THE BLACK EYED PEAS ♪♫♪

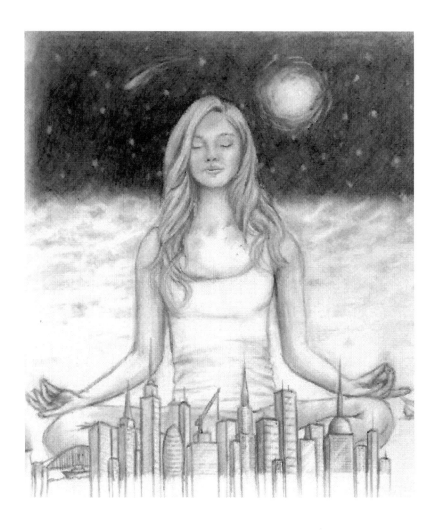

ARTWORK BY CRAIG DAWSON

Isn't it? Okay, so maybe not weirdos, but it is kind of that cool, Zen thing to do that I associate with health freaks and people with a lot of time on their hands. It's one of those things you try because it's supposed to chill you out, but then you find it doesn't really work because your brain just doesn't shut up, so you give it up as a lost cause. Or is that just me?

Seriously though, meditation does have a bad rap. Many feel that while it may be good before yoga, it doesn't really have a place in normal, everyday life. And I cringe to say that I was one of those people not long ago.

The truth is, meditation can be of benefit to anyone, from 3 to 103. It is easy to learn and practise and doesn't take nearly as long as you may assume. So, what is meditation, and what's all the hype about?

The most powerful thing about meditation is that it decreases the chatter of your brain. It helps us to relax and de-stress and increases our self-awareness and concentration. It can minimise anxiety and depression by allowing you to recognise negative thoughts and feelings and deal with them. Doctors are even beginning to suggest meditation for patients suffering from stress-related issues (it's only taken them a few thousand years to get with the program).

While meditation is present in Buddhism, Islam, Hinduism, and Christianity, and is used to help attain spiritual enlightenment, you do not have to be religious to use it. When you meditate you don't just relax, you consciously control the wanderings of your brain and focus them on just one thing. This could be a religious aspect, but I use meditation simply to calm my noisy brain, decrease stress, and centre myself. Like anything, it's all how you take it.

When I first tried meditation, I thought you had to wipe your mind completely blank, and I know this is a misconception many hold. The only thing these 'meditation' sessions achieved was giving me nice high levels of failure. There is no way I was getting my brain bound, gagged, and silent for even 2 minutes together!

It was a Facebook post that eventually put me on the right track. A friend had shared a little video of how to master meditation - in the next two minutes. I thought it was just another sensationalised post but got sucked into watching it anyway as you do with Facebook... And it was awesome! It focused on the one thing I'd always struggled with - clearing your mind. Turns out you're not even supposed to clear your mind! You're supposed to focus it. On just one thing. And that little piece of knowledge was all I needed to succeed with meditation.

When you meditate you aren't trying to switch off your brain, you're trying to narrow its focus. Instead of your brain skipping and jumping through negative thoughts, to-do lists, and general busyness, you focus on just one thing. This could be breathing, counting, an affirmation, a spiritual thought, or a happy feeling. Whenever your mind wanders you bring it back to your focus and carry on.

Meditation is not a way of making your mind quiet. It is a way of entering into the quiet that is already there - buried under the 50,000 thoughts the average person thinks every day.
-DEEPAK CHOPRA-

YouTube is full of tutorials and guided meditations, ▶ and you can download free apps ▶ as well that will teach and guide you in meditation. You don't need to spend hours a day doing it either. You can start with just 2 minutes and work your way up to 10 or 20 if you have time. You can plan meditation for the same time each day, or you can use it spontaneously during lunch breaks, in between meetings or school runs, or whenever you have a quiet, uninterrupted moment.

☻ The regular practice of mindfulness meditation has also been shown to affect the brain's plasticity, increasing grey matter in the hippocampus, an area of the brain important for learning, memory, and emotion, and reducing grey matter in the amygdala, an area of the brain associated with stress and anxiety.[33]

It helps to have a clutter-free space in which to meditate, even if that's just the corner of your bedroom. But if you don't have any space that could be called calming, or you're doing meditation on the run, then don't stress. The main thing is that you do a little bit every day. Consistently doing 2 minutes of meditation every day wherever you find yourself is far more beneficial than doing an hour once a week in a yoga retreat.

One of the easiest and best-known meditation methods is counting breaths. You can start with just a couple of minutes and build up to as long as feels comfortable.

---

[33] https://blog.bufferapp.com/how-to-rewire-your-brains-for-positivity-and-happiness

Here's how to start:

- Sit cross legged on the floor or seated in a chair. Make sure your back is straight and rest your hands comfortably on your knees.

- Close your eyes and breath slowly and naturally.

- Now focus your attention on your breathing. Feel the air going in and out as you breathe. Whenever you get distracted just bring your mind back to your breathing.

- After each exhalation but before you breathe in, count silently: 'one' (inhale, exhale) etc., until you reach 'five,' then start again from 'one.'

- When you've finished, slowly loosen your focus and open your eyes.

You can also take an affirmation ✇ 1 and centre your meditation around it.

- Sit cross legged on the floor or seated in a chair. Make sure your back is straight and rest your hands comfortably on your knees.

- Close your eyes and breath slowly and naturally.

- Inhale and smile. Think 'I love myself' or another affirmation of your choice.

- Exhale and relax your smile. Let go of any negative response to your affirmation.

- Whenever your mind wanders bring it gently back to your affirmation.

- Repeat for as long as you like.

A third way of meditating is to do so to music. 2
This is especially helpful if you find it hard to find a quiet place or time to meditate. If you're hiding in your room while the kids play in the yard, then this may be a good one for you.

- Sit cross legged on the floor or seated in a chair. Make sure your back is straight and rest your hands comfortably on your knees.

- Put in your headphones and pick a calm melody, preferably without words.

- Close your eyes and breath slowly and naturally.

- Let the music flow through you and focus on the tune. If you find yourself easily distracted, then try focusing on your breathing instead.

- Each time your mind wanders bring it back to your breathing or the music.

- Breathe slowly and deeply for the duration of the song.

So there you have three simple ways to meditate. You don't need a lot of time, and you need zero experience. All you need is a willingness to try, and to be consistent.

* * *

RECAP

- Meditation can benefit anyone. It decreases the chatter of your brain, helps us relax and de-stress, and increases our self-awareness and concentration.

- When you meditate you're not supposed to clear your mind. You're supposed to focus it on just one thing. This could be breathing, counting, a piece of music, an affirmation or a happy feeling.

- Consistency is the key with meditation. It is better to do 2 minutes of meditation a day than an hour once a week.

- You don't need any experience to meditate, just a willingness to try. It is easy to learn and practice, can be done anywhere, and can take just 1 minute.

ACTION STEPS ✎

Do now:

- Choose a meditation type and give it a shot. Like right now. If you've got time to read, you have 2 minutes to meditate. It is literally that quick.

Plan to:

- Meditate at least once a day, every day. It doesn't have to be at the same time each day. If spontaneous times work better for you then that's fine. It's the consistency that counts.

- Consider downloading an app, or bookmark YouTube tutorials to help guide you in your meditation.

- Join a meditation group in your local gym or park. Health groups will often run things like this for free in green spaces.

Work towards:

- Increasing your meditation 'til you reach around 20 minutes a day.

LINKED TO

1. Say it Like You Mean it

2. Create a Song and Dance

BREATH AND POSE!

♪♫♪ YOU MAKE MY DREAMS COME TRUE — DARYL HALL & JOHN OATES ♪♫♪

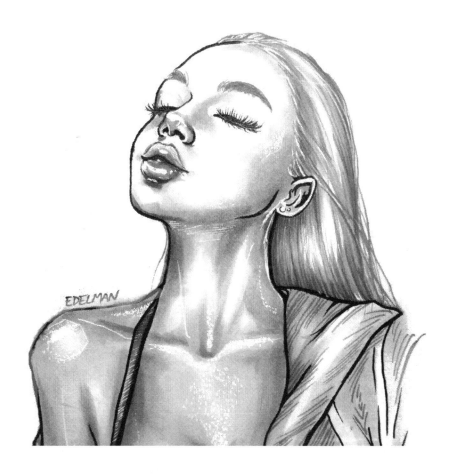

ARTWORK BY KELLY EDELMAN

> *"For breath is life, and if you breathe well you will live long on earth."*
> – SANSKRIT PROVERB-

Breathing. It's something we all do without a second thought. It's an automatic function of our body, and even when unconscious the body continues to breathe without any influence from us at all. And yet it is also the *only* autonomous system of the body that you can consciously control - if you know how.

Most of us never give a second thought to how we breathe - generally because we don't have to. We don't think of it as important. And yet when you start to focus on it, you realise that there is so much more you could be doing to optimize this function. We take around 23,000 breaths a day! That's a lot of opportunities to improve, and breathing properly can increase your energy, stamina, and quality of sleep. You actually know some of the ways in which breathing can help already, you just may not have connected the dots.

If you've had kids or even watched many mainstream comedy movies, then chances are you've heard about (and laughed at) the over-dramatized breathing pregnant woman are instructed to do during labour. 'Just breath through it' and 'deep breaths now.' Then there's victims of shock. 'Sit quietly and take deep slow breaths.' And what about when you're exercising? 'Breath evenly, you shouldn't be out of breath.' And if you've ever given yoga or meditation ✪1 a go then you'll know breathing is a huge part of both.

And yet somehow, we've never made the correlation between breathing consciously for certain aspects of our life and using breathing in *every* aspect of our lives. Not just occasionally, but every day, every hour, every minute! Which is an incredible waste, because **the way we breathe directly influences the way we feel, because breathing is closely tied to our emotions.**

When we are scared, angry, depressed or even frightened our breathing rhythm changes. It takes a bit of "breath awareness" to remember to breathe through powerful emotions.[34]

Breathing helps your mood by pumping endorphins into your system. Breathing deeply also actively cleanses and revitalizes the cells of your body. You can even 'breathe' your way out of negative feelings and pain. A friend of mine used breathing to help her with the pain and discomfort of getting a root canal. And put herself to sleep in the dentist chair!

Deep breathing is also called abdominal or belly breathing. It's done by inhaling slowly and deeply through your nose, causing your lungs to fill with air as your belly expands. Nose is the main word here. When we breathe through our nose the air is filtered and warmed for us.

Your mouth is for eating people - wait that didn't come out right... - I mean your mouth is for eating, people. (Oh, the importance of commas!)

---

[34] https://www.huffingtonpost.com/ornish-living/how-to-change-your-mood-w_b_6566412.html

"The nose is for breathing – the mouth is for eating."
– PROVERB -

Posture also plays a part in how we breathe and how we feel. I'm sure most of you have heard about the signals we inadvertently give to other people in the way we stand, hold our hands, and where we look. Well, not only do we give those signals to others with our posture, we give them to ourselves.

The expansion and release of your ribcage is what brings in oxygen - kind of like a big accordion. Sitting hunched over squashes your diaphragm and doesn't allow your lungs to expand fully. This alone has a big impact because it forces you to breathe shallowly; however, there is more at play than decreased breath. **Hunching and slouching literally make you feel smaller and less confident, and it's harder to think and act positively.** In contrast, standing or sitting with your head held high and shoulders back makes you look and feel more confident. It's easier to breathe and to regulate those breaths.

Think of your lungs as two big balloons. How hard would it be to blow a balloon up if someone was sitting on it? You wouldn't get much air in before it was whooshed right back out again. The same is true for bad posture. If you're hunched over it's almost impossible for your lungs to expand in the way they should, because your chest is restricted. Stand up straight, and hey presto! Your chest muscles can push outwards without restriction and your lungs can fill.

You know that feeling you get when you get home after a long day, take your bra off and throw it across the room? Okay, so maybe you don't but take my word for it - it's glorious! Why?

Because tight clothing like belts, bras, Spanx, and tight trousers hold your stomach and ribcage in, which means you can never draw a full breath. Not only is it uncomfortable, it's detrimental to your health! Even an overly muscled body can have the same effect - constricting the elasticity of your chest area.

And bonus! The quick shallow breaths that most of us take weaken our respiratory muscles, create tension in our upper body, and cause us to breath even more shallowly. Which can alter our posture, causing even more knock-on effects. So, if you're trying to suck your tummy in and breathe deeply at the same time - stop. It ain't gonna work!

⊛ Poor posture and breathing habits can also negatively affect how your body moves. Breathing from your chest instead of your belly causes a tightening in chest muscles which in turn cause rounded shoulders and a forward head posture. This causes your back to ache and your core strength to diminish. Interestingly, research has shown that people with chronic neck pain also show a reduction in respiratory function (they don't breathe as well as those without neck pain). It's all linked! [36]

When you first start standing and sitting up straight you'll probably get aching shoulders and back. This is your body re-aligning itself to how it should be. Sadly, your body has adapted to be more comfortable in the slumping position over the years. Don't be mistaken though, just because you're comfortable doesn't mean you're not doing a lot of harm to your body. The discomfort from sitting and standing correctly won't last forever, and you'll be well rewarded for your effort, so stick it out.

---

[36] http://rc.rcjournal.com/content/59/4/543

So, what's the solution? Well, obviously you need to improve your posture and your breathing, but habits of a lifetime are hard to break. I'm still working on these! Like anything, it is all about awareness. You know those pictures that have hidden elements which you can't find for the life of you, but then once you've seen it you can't un-see it? It's kind of like that. Now you know what you should be doing, you can correct yourself whenever you think of it.

Which, let's face it, is probably not going to be that often at first, so make it easy on yourself and set reminders. Set your phone to chime every hour and when it does, make a conscious effort to sit or stand up straighter, and breath deeper. It doesn't matter where you are or what you're doing, this is achievable. Breath and posture are easy to correct if you're consistent.

You might be in the middle of a meeting, cooking dinner, at your desk, or hanging washing. It doesn't matter. Roll your shoulders back, chest out, head up, and spine straight. Take deep slow breaths in and out through your nose. Hold this posture and concentrate on your breathing for as long as possible.

If you really want to get serious you could use athletic tape to hold your shoulders in the correct position. Ask a physiotherapist to do this for you the first time so you don't strap incorrectly. I would only bother with this if setting reminders is just not working or if your posture is already incredibly bad. Pilates, ballet, and yoga are also fabulous for working on your posture.

Here's a few other ways you can help your posture:

- Maintain a healthy weight. Excess weight, especially across your abdomen, weakens the stomach muscles, pulls the back muscles, and makes them work harder to keep you straight and tall.

- Exercise regularly⊘2. Not only does this help with excess weight, it tones your muscles and helps keep you flexible, so good posture becomes easier.

- Sleep in a good bed. Make sure your mattress supports your spine.

- Get your eyes checked. Hunching over to squint at your computer screen will not help your posture, so be sure to get your eyes checked regularly.

- Make sure everything fits you. Do your legs dangle off your chair? Get a footrest. Are you hunched over your desk? Look into standing workspaces or try stacking books under your computer screen if you can't spring for a new desk. Don't forget to adjust your car seat for good posture too!

- Think about your clothes. While skinny-legged jeans and bodysuits are making a comeback, make sure your fashion sense isn't impacting the way you walk, stand, or breathe. Tight bras, trousers, t-shirts, dresses, and suits can all inhibit your breathing and posture, so dress comfortably. The advent of spandex has helped a lot with this!

Breathing deeply and altering your posture are a fabulous help if you are angry, stressed, tired, anxious, or sad. It may not be by much, but it might be just enough to allow you to push through, try something else, or centre yourself. And sometimes that's all the help you need in that moment.

There are several different methods for improving your breathing, such as yogic breathing, Buteyko, Diaphragmatic breathing, and physical movement exercises. Each of these methods teach good breathing and posture techniques and they all come with a wealth of benefits outside of the mood ones we've discussed.

- Reduction in asthma symptoms and medication

- Reduction in allergic reactions

- Improvement in quality of life

- Increased stamina and energy

- Reduced nasal congestion

- Improved ability to cope with stress

- Reduction in anxiety or panic attacks

- Improved quality of sleep

- Reduction in snoring

- Improved thinking, learning and concentration levels

- Improved immunity and less susceptibility to colds and flu

- Improved ability to exercise and have enhanced sports performance

- Reduced tendency to headaches

All this from breathing! That's pretty flippin' good! Scientific research also shows breathing techniques can "improve patient reported outcomes and psychological state." So essentially - it doesn't matter what other treatments you're currently undertaking - breathing exercises will help. Here's a quick rundown on some of the methods.

Diaphragmatic breathing

This is a basic and simple breathing technique that maximizes air distribution in your lungs.

- You can lie down or sit.

- Concentrate on your breathing.

- Preferably you should breathe in slowly through your nose.

- When you inhale your abdomen should go out (not your chest).

- Exhale slowly with your abdomen going inward. Ideally exhalation (breathing out) should be twice as long as inhalation (breathing in).

Buteyko breathing

This is a program of breathing exercises, posture, and health and lifestyle guidelines to support a functional breathing pattern. The breathing exercises are designed to help normalise the breathing pattern and restore comfortable, natural nasal breathing.

- Sit upright, relax.

- Relax chest and belly muscles while breathing.

- Focus, close your eyes and look up.

- Breathe through your nose gently (keep mouth closed).

- Breath slowly and shallowly.

- Exhale slowly until you feel there is no air left in your lungs.

- Hold your breath as long as you can and then return to gentle breathing.

Physical movement exercises

- This type of breathing exercise combines physical elements and breathing elements.

- Focus on good posture.

- Relax (tense all muscles, and then relax, paying particular attention to muscles in shoulders and belly).

- Concentrate on breathing (close eyes). Focus on breathing while relaxed in rest position. Focus on breathing with shoulder rotation. Focus on breathing with forward curl. Focus on breathing with arm raises.

Yoga

When doing yoga you hold poses and concentrate on your breathing.

- Sit on a blanket in Sukhasana or Easy Cross-Legged Pose. Root your sit-bones and feel your spine grow long as you lightly extend from the crown of the head. Soften your heart and your shoulders.

- Place your hand over your navel and take a slow, deep breath into your belly. Feel the belly inflate like a balloon as you inhale and deflate as you exhale. Practice this for five breaths.

- Move your hand two to three inches above your navel to your rib cage. Feel the ribs expand as you inhale and retract as you exhale. Practice this for five breaths.

- Place your hand below your collarbone, at the centre of your chest, and inhale. Feel the chest spread as you breathe in and withdraw on an exhale. Practice this for five breaths.

See how important breathing is! And you thought it was just keeping you alive. While I concede that may be the most important function of breathing, the quality of that life is incredibly important too. And by simply learning how to breathe and position your body properly, you will increase your mood and your health. Beautifully simple!

* * *

RECAP ✄

- Breathing is the only autonomous system of the body that you can consciously control.

- Breathing properly can increase your energy, stamina, and quality of sleep. It also directly influences the way we feel, by pumping endorphins into your system.

- Posture also plays a part in how we breathe and how we feel. Hunching and slouching literally make you feel smaller and less confident, and it's harder to think and act positively. Your lungs can't expand the way they should because your chest is restricted.

- Luckily breath and posture are easy to correct if you're consistent. Start by standing tall and taking deep breaths through your nose every time you think of it. Both of these things are also are great help when you're feeling angry, stressed, tired, anxious or sad.

ACTION STEPS ✎

Do now:

- Look at how you're sitting or standing. How could it be improved? Try altering your posture for the better and for the worse. Sit up straight with shoulders back and head help high. Breathe deeply through your nose, letting your belly fill and expand. Say an affirmation to yourself. How do you feel? Do you believe the affirmation?

- Now slump. Curve your back, let your shoulders roll forward and drop your head. Breathe shallowly through your mouth. Say an affirmation to yourself. How do you feel? Do you believe the affirmation? Do the two positions feel different?

Plan to:

- Set reminders to help you focus on and remedy your posture and breathing.

- Begin to use both breathing and posture when your emotions are running high as a first line of defence.

- Practice good breathing and posture exercises each day.

Work towards:

- Having good posture and breathing techniques the majority of the time without any reminders.

- Using breathing and posture to combat high emotion times both consciously and subconsciously.

LINKED TO 🔗

1. Meditation is for Weirdos

2. Exercise Your Mind

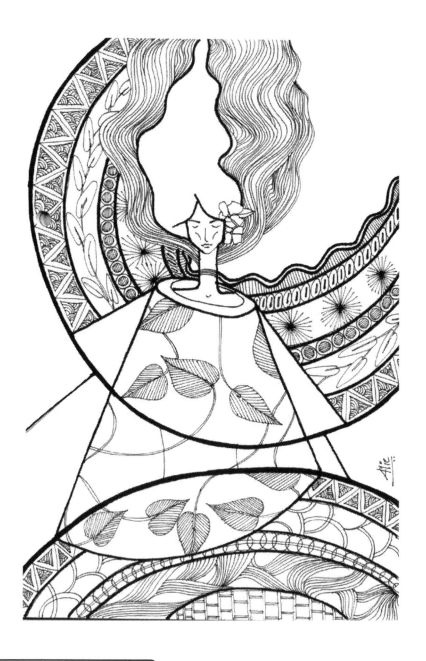

ARTWORK BY 4LIE_ARTWORKS

BODY

YOUR BODY AND YOUR MIND ARE INTRINSICALLY LINKED, AND NOT JUST BECAUSE YOUR MIND DIRECTS YOUR BODY. BUT BECAUSE WHAT YOU FEED YOUR BODY, HOW YOU MOVE, AND THE SITUATIONS YOU SUBJECT YOUR BODY TO, HAVE A PROFOUND IMPACT ON YOUR MIND AND FROM THERE YOUR MOOD.

EAT THE FOOD!

♪♫♪ CHICKEN FRIED — ZACH BROWN ♪♫♪

"One cannot think well, love well,
sleep well, if one has not dined well."
- VIRGINIA WOOLF -

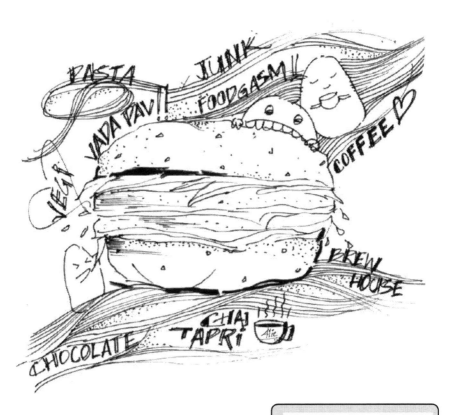

ARTWORK BY 4LIE_ARTWORKS

I know a lot about healthy food. It's something that fascinates me. I know how something that can be really beneficial for one person can act like a poison to another. I know what types of things we're eating too much of as a society, and what we need to eat more of. But one thing that I didn't know until a couple of years ago is how much of an impact the food we put into our bodies has on our brains.

One of the most famous quotes about the benefit of healthy food on your body comes from the Greek physician Hippocrates, and while I'm sure you've heard it, it's something many of us have forgotten in a world where we can pick up pills for weight loss, headaches, heartburn, and coughs.

"Let food be thy medicine, and medicine be thy food."
— HIPPOCRATES -

Hippocrates is referred to as 'the father of modern medicine,' and he was a smart cookie. He knew that a healthy diet rich in vitamins and minerals was, and still is, a great way to prevent many ailments, and far better for you than simply taking a pill to fix the symptoms of ill health.

I think as a society we are always looking for the 'quick fix,' the easy way out, and our bodies and brains are suffering as a result of this. The busier and more stressed we get, the harder the body has to work, and without the nourishment it needs, your body malfunctions, and struggles to maintain good health.

And **if your body is suffering then so is your brain.** You see, the brain draws its energy and sustenance from the body. If your body is run down and unhealthy, then by default your brain will suffer too. And a brain in pain sure as heck doesn't make you happy! I'm not saying low mood can be fixed or prevented just by eating well, but it sure as hell helps!

It is becoming increasingly obvious that food plays a massive role in the healthy function of our brain, and from there, our moods. My daughter and I both get 'hangry.' You know, angry when we're hungry (well, I get irritable). This happens because your brain takes 20% of the energy we gain from our food to function. And what does the brain do? It controls our thoughts, our actions, and our moods. And if we're not eating good food, then the brain suffers.

Good food = Healthy brain = Happy mood

Some of the most important things for a healthy mind can only be obtained through what you put in your mouth. They can't be made in the body. This means when you run low, your body suffers. Sometimes your body tries to borrow what it needs from other areas, which then spreads the negative effects, so it is incredibly important to keep replenishing everything the body needs to function, not just well, but spectacularly!

> *"Foods rich in vitamins, minerals, and fatty acids are not only super healthy, but can also increase happiness, lessen symptoms of depression, and quell anxiety."*[37]

The processed foods that make up many people's diets are high in sodium, starches, bulking agents, and preservatives, and don't provide your body with much in the way of goodness. I'm

---

[37] www.greatist.com/happiness/nutrients-boost-mood

not going to tell you to minimize processed foods. You already know that. The sugar alone in most packaged foods is huge, and sugar truly does live up to its nickname of 'The White Death.' Studies are beginning to link high sugar intake to depression, and it also causes high blood pressure, energy slumps, and general ill health, amongst a raft of other things!

> ☢ The most common nutritional deficiencies seen in patients with mood disorders according to research published by the NCBI[38] are of omega–3 fatty acids, B vitamins, minerals, and the amino acids that are precursors to neurotransmitters like the all-important serotonin. And our SAD (standard American Diet) is the major culprit.

But like I said, you already know this. So instead of focusing on what not to eat, we're going to talk about what you *should* be eating.

Many of us studied healthy eating in school, or have watched documentaries since, but how many of us remember what we're supposed to be eating, and (here's the kicker) actually do it! What's healthy has had several revamps over the years as new knowledge has come to light, but the basic premise has stayed the same.

We should eat a wide variety of colourful vegetables, legumes and fruits every day. Around 5 serves of vegetables and 2 of fruit. (A serve is roughly the size of your hand). Healthy whole grains and cereals, and either lean meat, poultry, fish, eggs, legumes, and beans should be eaten with every meal. Add milk, yoghurt and cheese, or their alternatives in small quantities

---

[38] https://www.ncbi.nlm.nih.gov/pmc/articles/PMC2738337/

along with healthy fats such as olive oil, avocado, seeds, and nuts.

How much you eat of each category is largely based on how much you move, your age and gender, and your cultural background. There are calculators online which will help you work this out. Did you know that Asians metabolise beans better than anyone else? Or that Africans have the highest dairy sensitivity in the world? Cool, huh!

Always eat food whole and unprocessed where possible (a piece of fruit instead of fruit juice, porridge oats instead of sugar filled cereal, baked potato instead of hot chips). Try eating low GI foods (slow release energy) so you reach for snacks less. Branch out and try new things. Variety is the spice of life, and eating healthy certainly doesn't have to be boring!

> ☻ "Low glycaemic index (GI) foods such as some fruits and vegetables, whole grains, pasta, etc. are more likely to provide a moderate but lasting effect on brain chemistry, mood, and energy level than the high GI foods" [39]

That's the (very) brief overview anyway. Now let's look a bit closer at a few things.

Carbohydrates

Society has villainized carbohydrates to the point where we think of them as 'bad' or a 'sometimes food,' but in actual fact they are incredibly important for the whole body's health. I love the quote from the movie 'The Holiday' where Cameron Diaz's character says, 'I want to eat carbs, without wanting to kill

---

[39] https://www.ncbi.nlm.nih.gov/pmc/articles/PMC2738337/

myself!' This is how many people feel about carbs, and diets like Atkins and Dukan sure didn't help.

Carbs break down into glucose in your body and provide fuel for our brain, most of our organs, and our bodies while exercising. I mean, it doesn't get much more important than that. And yet we are limiting them!

People following a low-carb diet often find themselves fatigued, lethargic, and with low mood, something I encountered firsthand. I went on an almost zero carb diet to lose baby weight after the birth of my daughter. I felt great at first, and I definitely lost weight, but after a while I found myself running out of steam and becoming more and more irritable.

I ended up with adrenal fatigue, and a constant string of illnesses, and I also think being extremely low carb played a huge role in my spiral from sadness to depression. Many of these things had other contributing factors, of course, but low carb definitely played its part. I cannot emphasise enough - your body needs carbs!

Don't get me wrong, those highly processed carbs full of sugar and sodium are defiantly bad, but there is a plethora of healthy alternatives. Whole grains, fruits, vegetables, and legumes are all great choices, and also bring fibre and other nutrients to the party. Eating carbs helps boost your tryptophan levels (a non-essential amino acid), which in turn helps synthesize serotonin, one of the 'happy chemicals,' which lifts your mood.

Sometimes we limit carbs unintentionally for health reasons. I still have to be careful I'm getting enough good carbs in my diet, because my gluten sensitivity leaves me vomiting and exhausted if I get even a trace, but I am so much luckier than people 10 years ago. There are more gluten free and generally healthy carbohydrate alternatives readily available now than there ever has been before. Spelt, Quinoa, Buckwheat, and Amaranth are all fabulous alternatives to wheat and are delicious too. Honest. You should be able to find healthy carb alternatives no matter what your dietary requirements are.

Start adding healthy carbs in the form of whole fruits and vegetables, whole grains, and legumes into your diet a little at a time. Roughly 50% of your plate should be carbohydrates at each meal. If this sounds scary or if you have been low carb for a long time, then just start slowly and increase over time.

I will never cut carbs out of my diet again, and I encourage you not to either. They are just too important!

Low GI Foods

I mentioned low GI foods briefly above, but many people, while they've heard the term, don't actually know what they are. GI stands for Glycaemic Index, which is simply a ranking of the carbohydrates in your food according to how they affect your blood glucose levels.

☢ Carbohydrates with a low GI value (55 or less) are more slowly digested, absorbed, and metabolised, and cause a lower and slower rise in blood glucose and, therefore usually, insulin levels. [40] Replacing those high-glycaemic foods with low-glycaemic choices will assist in getting a slow, sustained release of insulin that keeps your blood sugar levels even, followed by a gradual rise in serotonin. No rapid rise and no rapid crash of serotonin levels means you have an even mood all day. [41]

---

[40] https://www.gisymbol.com/about-glycemic-index/
[41] http://www.healthmates.com.au/blog/low-glycemic-foods

When you skip meals, eat sugary snacks or drinks, or eat highly processed foods (all high GI), your blood glucose levels spike and then crash. This means you get that lovely boost of energy quickly, but it's then followed by tiredness, crankiness, and decreased mental function. Which means you grab another coffee/bagel/biscuit and the rollercoaster ride begins again. If you drew it, it would look like a zig zagged line with lots of peaks and lows.

Low GI carbs, on the other hand, are digested and released slowly, which gives your body sustained energy. This would look like a straight line. Nice and even with no peaks and lows.

A few low GI examples are oats, quinoa, bulgur wheat, long grain rice, whole wheat spaghetti, soy milk, lima beans, and peanuts. Most non-starchy vegetables are low GI too, which makes things easy, and tomatoes, cherries, peaches, apples, pears, grapes, and oranges are as well.

A low GI diet has been linked not only to improvements in mood, but in blood sugar and insulin control, disease prevention, and an increase in energy (always helpful). This is why it's not just crucial to have carbohydrates in your diet, but to choose the right ones.

Fats

Fat, glorious fat! Your grandmother has it right when she says, 'Fat is flavour.' It's why most people prefer chicken thigh to chicken breast, proper gravy over instant, and butter over margarine. It just tastes better! Fat also has the power to lift our emotional state and reduce feelings of hunger.

And yet most of us are still actively trying to cut fat out of our diets because we have been told it is bad and the root of all our weight issues. And if you're talking about artificial fats such as vegetable oil, then yes, it is.

But there are stacks of amazing natural fats that are incredibly important for our bodies and brains. Avocados, olive oil, coconut oil, grass-fed beef, butter, nuts and seeds, and omega 3's from fish, are some of the goodies. Every meal we eat should have a small portion of healthy fat included. **Good fats boost brain function, help lower bad cholesterol and raise the good, and prevent against belly fat.** They even help you poo well!

Of your total daily calories only 25-30% should come from fat. So, the average person should consume between 40 and 85 grams of fat per day depending on their age, gender, and level of activity. And of that amount, only a third should be saturated fat (think meat, dairy products, coconut oil). The rest of your fat intake should be from unsaturated fats (think seafood, nuts and seeds, olive oil, and avocados).

Trans fat intake (think doughnuts, margarine, vegetable oil, most processed foods) should be ZERO. Yup, that trans fat is bad news!

> ☢ Trans fats are unsaturated fats that have been processed and as a result, behave like saturated fats. Eating trans fats increases the levels of 'bad' cholesterol and decreases the levels of 'good' cholesterol in the body, which is a major risk factor for heart disease. It is important to lower the amounts of trans fats you eat to help you stay healthy.[42]

---

[42] https://www.eatforhealth.gov.au/food-essentials/fat-salt-sugars-and-alcohol/fat

Processed food that contains little to no fat normally has a stack of sugar to give you the same flavour and satiety. It also doesn't keep you as full for as long, which means you're rummaging for food again sooner than you would be if you'd just eaten the fat in the first place.

Here's some examples of what could make up your daily fat intake:

- Almonds- 23 nuts: 14g fat

- Walnuts (chopped)- 1/4 cup: 18g fat

- Avocado- ½ avocado: 15g fat

- Olive Oil- 1 tablespoon: 14g fat

- Peanut Butter (smooth)- 1 tablespoon: 8g fat

- Olives (green or black)- 8 jumbo olives: 5g fat

- Sunflower Seeds (unsalted, roasted, hulled)- 1/4 cup: 16g fat

- Butter, salted- 1 tablespoon: 12g fat.

- Beef roast- 120g: 12g fat

- Egg (1 large): 5g fat

- Salmon fillet: 6g fat

- Milk- 1 cup: 8g fat

So, you see, it really does help to know your fats. Some have beneficial properties, and others detrimental. But your body definitely needs it, so stop villainizing fat and start eating it. Make sure it's good quality, natural fat, and have it in small amounts, but get into it!

Omega-3 Fatty Acids

We're going to take a closer look at omega-3 fatty acids, because they are one of the most important 'brain foods' there are. I'm sure you've heard of them before. They are part of all cell membranes in the body and are necessary for a healthy brain and nervous system. Omega-3's reduce inflammation, the risk of heart disease, improve your hair, skin, and nails, and your mental health. Our hunter gatherer ancestors ate 5-10 times more omega-3 than us, and they not only survived, but they evolved into a stronger, more mentally adept primate.

Omega-3s are found predominately in salmon, and other oily fish such as mackerel, tuna, sardines, and bluefish. Now I don't know about you, but I've never eaten mackerel or bluefish in my life. It's too expensive to buy, and we don't own a boat. Salmon, sardines, and tuna, however, are available pretty much everywhere, and the canned varieties are even quite cheap.

There is no 'official' recommendation for omega-3 intakes, but USDA Dietary Guidelines for Americans 2010 suggests healthy adults consume 250 milligrams of omega-3 fatty acids each day, for a total of 1,750 milligrams per week. Others say 500 mg a day is better. Honestly, just start. Anything is better than nothing, and while you can aim for 500 a day, don't beat yourself up if you don't get there. And don't stress, 500 mg might sound like a lot but it's only half a gram!

While fresh fish is always better, canned fish still contains decent amounts of omega-3s. An 85 g (3-ounce) serving of salmon gives you 1.1-1.9 g of omega-3s. A 95 g (3.35 ounces) tin of salmon gives you pretty much the same, 1.5-2 g of omega-3s, whereas a 95 g can of tuna only has around 0.1-0.4 of a gram. That's a big difference, so if you're not a fan of salmon you're going to have to eat a lot more of other things!

Salmon also provides more calcium and has less methylmercury than tuna, with sardines also containing only a small amount. (This is only something you really need to worry about if you are pregnant, giving a lot of fish to a small child, or eating a lot yourself!)

> ☻ "Healthy brains and nerve cells depend on omega-3s because the nervous system is made mostly of fat. The signals that travel through our flesh — feelings, thoughts, commands to our bodies — skip along cells and their arms sheathed in fat. Brain cell membranes are about 20 percent fatty acids and they seem to be crucial for keeping brain signals moving smoothly".[43]

If you're not a fan of fish, or if you're a vegetarian or vegan, try flaxseeds, chia seeds, and hemp seeds. They all have good levels of omega-3s. Dark leafy greens such as spinach and romaine provide small amounts, as do mung beans and cauliflower.

The biggest problem with trying to get your omega-3 intake from plants is that they don't contain it in nearly as high amounts as marine-based omega-3s. They also tend to have high amounts of omega-6, which is what your omega-3s are trying to balance in the first place.

Kale, olive oil, and walnuts, are plant-based sources that are often recommended for omega-3 intake, and while they do contain some, their high levels of omega-6 make them pretty worthless.

---

[43] https://www.psychologytoday.com/us/articles/200301/omega-3s-boosting-mood

The nutritional data website[44] will give you a rundown of which foods have the highest levels of omega-3, but if you want to keep it simple just try to eat seafood 2-3 times a week, even if it's out of a can. Not only will it boost your mood, but it will help prevent heart disease, build a healthy brain, and protect against cancer.

Fruit and Vegetables

This shouldn't come as a shock to anyone. We need lots of fruit and veg in our diets. Well, lots of veg and a couple of serves of fruit. Vegetables in general are pretty awesome, but some are simply better than others. (Sorry, potato, but you're just not that great.) Dark green leafy vegetables, for example, are a powerhouse of nutrients. 'Greens' like iceberg lettuce, on the other hand, have very little in the way of beneficial nutrients (it's more white if you really think about it anyway...).

Green smoothies have become all the rage in recent years and with good reason! Dark green leafy vegetables have so many health benefits it's ridiculous. Did you know kale has almost as much vitamin C as an orange? And that leafy greens are also an important source of vitamin B, B3, B6, and B9? (Animal foods such as shellfish and beef are the only naturally occurring sources of B12).

Our 'greens' are also a fabulous source of folate. And what does folate do? Contributes to serotonin development, which as I'm sure you know by now, helps lift your mood. Spinach, chard, and other dark leafy greens also contain magnesium, which can positively impact serotonin levels and boost your mood. (Pumpkin seeds, Brazil nuts, chickpeas, and beans are also rich in magnesium).

---

[44] http://nutritiondata.self.com/foods-000140000000000000000.html

> *"The B vitamins are needed to make many neurotransmitters, and the B's have long been considered anti-stress vitamins.*[45]

If you struggle to get enough greens into your diet, then I recommend reading the book *Green Smoothie Detox* by Kylie Ansett.▶ It shows you how to create amazing smoothies that taste great and make you feel fabulous! My whole family likes these green smoothies and they have several serves of fruit and veg in each one. Bonus - they keep up to 4 days, so you can pre-make them, stick them in a travel cup, and run out the door with it.

Another great way to get additional greens in your diet (or your picky child's) is to add them to meat dishes as a 'filler.' I use zucchini in meat patties in place of breadcrumbs, kale in bolognaise, and add vegetables to all my curries and bakes. Not only does it taste great, it helps balance out the meat in a meal, and provides me with those veg serves my body needs.

Veggies do not have to be boring! Try different spices and sauces in stir-fries or create fun veg meals like stuffed capsicums. Get your kids involved and make racing cars and faces out of cucumber and carrots, broccoli, beans, and cauliflower. The ideas are endless! Try cutting up raw vegs and leaving them in the fridge as a snack box. That way when you reach for a fast snack you've got one all ready to go.

Fruit is also a fabulous snack. It provides sugars, fibre, water, and carbs along with vitamins, minerals, and antioxidants, in

---

[45] https://www.livestrong.com/slideshow/557976-foods-that-can-improve-your-mood/#slide=10

one simple package (if you eat it whole). Much of this is lost when you consume fruit as juice, so keep it whole and you're good to go! Fruit is also quite filling, so if you're snacking on fruit you're automatically going to be snacking less on other things.

Berries of all kinds usually make it to the top of any brain foods list too. They are bursting with flavonoids, which protect your brain from damage and play a role in improving cognitive skills, such as learning, memory, and decision making. Berries have also been linked with having a more positive mood. Yee ha! So fruit (especially berries) and vegetables (especially leafy greens) are a must every day.

Protein

20% of the human body is made up of protein, and it plays a crucial role in almost all biological processes. Protein in turn is made up of strings of amino acids, and a large proportion of our muscles, cells, and tissues are made up of these. It can also act as an energy source when glucose is low! So, kind of important... But here's the kicker. Only 11 of the 20 essential amino acids are manufactured by our body. The remaining 9 have to be supplied through diet.

Serious physical and mental health issues can arise from a lack of essential amino acids in the body. [46]

Unlike with fats and carbohydrates, the body doesn't store amino acids. The proteins in our bodies are constantly being

---

[46] http://www.thenourishedpsychologist.com/protein-and-mental-health/

broken down and replaced. That's why it's so important to have a small portion of protein at every meal or snack to replenish them. (Yet another reason why protein balls became so popular).

Protein helps keep your energy up, and your blood sugar stable. Replacing the depleted amino acids through complete protein (those proteins containing all the essential amino acids we need), can also boost feelings of well-being and vitality, and positively affect brain functionality and your mental health! Yup, pretty important. So, if you're not great at adding protein to your meals, then this is something you're going to have to work on!

> ☢ The entire amino acid pool is transformed, or 'exchanged' three to four times a day. This means that the body has to be supplied with more amino acids, partly by protein biosynthesis, partly by the diet or through consumption of suitable dietary supplements. [47]

A high-quality balanced diet naturally contains all the essential amino acids. Only problem is, most of us don't eat a high-quality balanced diet... Eggs, milk, yogurt, seafood, cheese, turkey, beef, pork, and chicken are all excellent sources of amino acids and are considered complete proteins. In fact, the only animal protein that isn't a complete protein is gelatin. It's missing one. Roughly 75% of the protein we eat in our diets should be complete or high-quality protein.

---

[47] http://www.aminoacid-studies.com/amino-acids/what-are-amino-acids.html

*A complete protein is one that
contains all of the essential amino
acids in quantities sufficient for
growth and repair of body tissue.* [48]

But if you're not a big meat eater, have a dairy sensitivity, or abstain for religious, ethical, or health reasons, then this becomes a bit tricky because plant proteins usually lack at least one amino acid. But it's not impossible.

Whole grains, lentils, chickpeas, black beans, pinto beans, almonds, walnuts, and sunflower seeds are all rich in essential amino acids - although none of them contain them all. They have to be combined with other plant proteins to get the complete profile. Baked beans on toast is a great example of combining plant-based proteins.

Protein powders, while not as good as whole foods, do contain a high number of the essential proteins. These are generally listed on the label under an 'essential amino acid profile,' making it easy to see what you need to add.

Vegetables in generous amounts can also provide a surprisingly high percentage of amino acids.

Soy products, quinoa, and Amaranth (the seed of a leafy green), are stand out winners if you're trying to avoid animal protein. They contain all 9 of the essential amino acids without having to worry about combining. So do hemp seeds, pumpkin seeds, and buckwheat. And bonus - they're all gluten free!

---

[48] https://www.encyclopedia.com/science-and-technology/biochemistry/biochemistry/amino-acid

So how much should you eat? Well, like most things - not as much as we do! Remember that the body can't store protein. So, while you may need to eat it frequently, you don't need a lot. I'm talking to you, Atkins and Dukan. Any protein we consume that is over and above what our body needs is stored as fat. Yup - fat. So, while gorging on pulled pork or Korean BBQ is incredibly tasty, it's going straight to your fat stores! It's not just our waistline that suffers either. Our kidneys are also left working overtime, getting rid of all the ammonia caused by the body's breakdown of the excess protein.

An easy way to calculate the amount of protein you should eat each day is to multiply your body weight in kilograms by 0.8 or in pounds by 0.36. This means a 68-kg/150-pound person should eat around 54 grams of protein a day. Pregnant women and those who are physically active need a bit more, and of course this is just a rough guideline. Everyone is different. Here's what 54 grams of protein looks like.

- A 28 gram (1 ounce) piece of meat or skinless poultry contains around 7 grams of **complete** protein when cooked.

- Peanut butter contains 7 grams of protein per TBSP.

- An egg also has around 7 grams of **complete** protein.

- A 100 gram (3.5 ounce) fillet of Atlantic salmon has a little more than 22 grams of **complete** protein per ounce cooked.

- 1 cup of tinned red kidney beans gives you 12 grams of protein.

- 1 cup of yogurt varies between 8 and 12 grams of **complete** protein.

- ¼ cup of almonds gives you 8 grams of protein.

- 1 cup of milk contains 8 grams of **complete** protein.

- Hemp seeds (or hulled hemp hearts) contain 10 grams of **complete** protein for every 2 TBSP consumed.

- 28 grams (1 ounce) of cheese has between 6grams (soft cheese) and 10grams (hard cheese) of **complete** protein.

- Pumpkin seeds (pepitas) have 10 grams of **complete** protein per ¼ cup serve.

- Amaranth has 9 grams of **complete** protein per 1 cup serve.

- Quinoa has 8 grams of **complete** protein per 1 cup serve.

- A 170 gram (6 ounce) can of tuna has 40 grams of **complete** protein.

- Buckwheat has 6 grams of **complete** protein per 1 cup serve.

So as with all things, when it comes to protein - moderation is key. But eat it at every meal if you can. And make sure it's complete protein. Or if it's not, do a food combo with another incomplete protein to fill in the gaps. Clear as mud? Awesome. Let's move on!

Fluids

Coffee, tea (my weakness), and carbonated beverages, are high in caffeine, something I'm sure you already knew. But did you know caffeine is bad for anxiety, agitation, and depression? You did, but you still love it? Well, did you know it can also keep you awake at night, which has the knock-on effect of making you tired, irritable, and more prone to mood swings? Hot chocolate also has caffeine, and while the milk is great before bed, the chocolate itself will not help your sleep!

Carbonated drinks are also incredibly bad for you - and even more so for woman. Research shows that high cola consumption has been linked to an increase in fractures in young women, and a lower bone density - something which used to only affect the elderly. The high sugar content in most carbonated drinks just adds to this issue. Carbonated water has so far proven to be safe.

Alcohol. What can I say? It's bad for your mood and your health. You had to have seen that coming. Don't get me wrong, the first few drinks might make you feel good, but alcohol has a depressant effect. This means after the buzz has worn off, you will be left feeling even more down than before. So, steer clear if you suffer from recurring mood issues or have just one drink occasionally.

If you find yourself reaching for alcohol more often than you should, have a closer look. Why are you drinking? Is it because you enjoy it, or because it's simply a habit, or are you trying to cover something else up? Alcohol dependence is a bigger problem now than ever before - especially among those with low mood. You might think you only have a drink when you've had a bad day, but how many bad days have you had this week? If you think alcohol is becoming a problem, seek help.

If you want to go out drinking with your mates, try matching a glass of water with every glass of alcohol. This will help keep your blood alcohol down, cut your total number of drinks in half, and bonus - cost you far less

So what drinks does that leave us? Well, plain old water still wins the fluid race hands down. Pure water helps hydrate your body and flushes out toxins and wastes. And most people are not getting enough of it. Dehydration happens more frequently than you might think, and one of the warning signs? Fatigue. So instead of grabbing a coffee or a cola when you're sleepy, try a glass of water. You might just need a top up!

Green tea and other herbal teas can also be beneficial as they provide antioxidants without the caffeine or sugar, and green smoothies are a powerhouse of nutrition. Everything else needs to be a sometimes drink. Sorry.

Chocolate

Here's something you're going to enjoy. **Chocolate helps with low mood!** But before you race off to the pantry for your milk chocolate, let's talk specifics.

Dark chocolate (70% cocoa solids or more) is a great source of tryptophan (the sleep promotor), and the anti-stress mineral magnesium. It is also one of the few dietary sources of anandamide, a naturally occurring neurotransmitter called the *"bliss molecule."*

"Chocolate contains phenylethylamine which can raise levels of endorphins, the pleasure-giving substances, in the brain"
-PSYCHOLOGIST SUE WRIGHT-

Researchers found that chocolate melted on the tongue (this seems to be the key) raised the heart rate, and all areas of the brain were boosted with a buzz that lasted four times longer than a passionate kiss. This explains why people can become addicted to it. Of course, chocolate in large amounts makes you fat, whereas kissing can have the opposite effect...

Chocolate also contains caffeine, which has a stimulatory effect on the brain, so don't eat it before bed. This includes that late cup of hot chocolate.

Dark chocolate has even been shown to reduce food cravings, whereas milk chocolate raises them. Look for at least 70% on the label. The higher the percentage the better it is for you. I really enjoy 70%, whereas a 90% chocolate from Lindt (who makes amazing choccie!) sat in my fridge for months because it was just too bitter for me to enjoy.

And we're not talking about half a block here either. 1.5-3 ounces (42-85 grams) is all you need. Roughly 4 squares of Lindt 70% or 8 squares of Cadbury 70%. Now all I need to do is find a scientific study telling me Scotch is healthy, and I'll be golden!

A few more goodies

- Eggs are one of the easiest to metabolize foods in the world. They are high in tryptophan, the building block amino acid for serotonin, and have a lot of good cholesterol. The Heart Foundation gave them a bad rap for a few years, but it was all a misunderstanding, and they've recently given them the tick of approval. Protein-rich eggs also include amino acids and essential fatty acids.

- Probiotics, whether from supplements or foods, are beneficial for more than digestive health. People who take probiotics see improvements in their perceived levels of stress and have a more positive mental outlook compared to people not taking probiotics.

- Vitamin C has been shown to reduce cortisol (the stress hormone). High levels of vitamin C are found in hot chillies and bell peppers as well as raw fruits like oranges, cantaloupe, papayas, and kiwi.

Weight loss and mood

Unfortunately, when we're feeling down we tend to gravitate towards comfort foods. Those sugary, starchy, highly processed foods that don't provide our body with much in the way of nutrition. Those foods that cause us to stockpile weight and move less. All these things keep you feeling rubbish, which makes you crave comfort food more. It's a vicious cycle. Craving sugar can also be a warning sign for depression. It gives you a temporary high, but then you crash and come back for more. Essentially people with low mood make bad food choices, which then cripples their health even more.

Healthy foods, on the other hand, help with slow and steady weight loss. They feed our body and our brain and create a lift in mood and energy. We are more inspired to eat better as a result. Data shows there is a strong link between healthy weight loss and a lift in mood. Who doesn't like seeing a slimmer, healthier image in the mirror? Careful weight loss through healthy eating (not fad diets), can help break that vicious cycle, and lift both your body image and your mood.

Eating is not all about the food though. Mealtimes themselves can be a time to de-stress, recharge, and connect 🔗 1 with other people. They shouldn't be a rushed moment where you shove food into your mouth, but a positive experience that nourishes us mentally and physically. I'm a shocker at this. I often turn up to school pickup with fruit in my hand because I've missed lunch. It's something I'm actively working on because while I've managed to cut caffeinated tea from my diet and include healthier options to my meals, set mealtimes is the thing that constantly trips me!

Eating regular meals, especially breakfast, has been shown to increase your energy, memory, and mood, and help with a balanced weight. The old adage from Adelle Davis that goes, "Eat breakfast like a King, lunch like a Prince, and dinner like a pauper," is as true now as the day she coined it. A good breakfast to start the day would include some lean protein, good fats, and healthy carbohydrates. How many of us get all that in our breakfast?

Bottom line? Diet alone cannot combat low mood. But healthy diet changes can bring about changes in our brain structure, which in turn can help lift mood. So, eat your healthy carbs, increase your omega-3, consider adding things like healthy fats and green smoothies to your diet, and see what a difference it can make to your body, and your brain.

* * *

RECAP 📌

- It is becoming increasingly obvious that food plays a massive role in the healthy function of our brain, and from there, our moods. How? The brain draws its energy and sustenance from the body. If your body is run down and unhealthy, then by default your brain will suffer too.

- Some of the most important things for a healthy mind can only be obtained through what you put in your mouth. They can't be made by the body. This is why eating a broad range of healthy food is so important.

- Processed foods are high in sugar, sodium, starches, bulking agents and preservatives, and don't provide your body with much in the way of goodness. Studies are beginning to link high sugar intake to depression, as well as high blood pressure, energy slumps, and general ill health.

- Carbohydrates are incredibly important for our whole bodies' health. They provide fuel for our brain, most of our organs, and our bodies while exercising. Whole grains, fruits, vegetables, and legumes are all examples of healthy carbs.

- Good fats boost brain function, help lower bad cholesterol and raise the good, and prevent against belly fat. They also help you feel fuller for longer.

- Omega-3 fatty acids are one of the most important brain foods there are. They reduce inflammation, and the risk of heart disease, improve your hair, skin, and nails and boost your mental health. They are found predominantly in salmon and other oily fish but can also be found in flaxseeds, chia seeds, and hemp seeds.

- Leafy greens are an important source of B vitamins and folate, and many also contain magnesium. Magnesium and folate both have a positive impact on serotonin levels which in turn boosts your mood.

- 20% of the human body is made up of protein, and it plays a crucial role in almost all biological processes. The body doesn't store the amino acids protein is made up of which is why it's important to eat a small amount of protein with every meal.

- Dark chocolate is a great source of tryptophan (the sleep promotor) and the anti-stress mineral magnesium.

- Caffeine is bad for anxiety, agitation and depression. Alcohol also has a depressant effect, which means after the buzz has worn off you will be left feeling even more down than before.

- People with low mood make bad food choices which then cripples their health even more. Making small changes consistently can help feed our body and brain and create a lift in mood and energy.

ACTION STEPS ✎

Do now:

- Think back to the last 3 meals you ate. What were they? Would they win praise from health critics or leave them horrified?

- Write down the top 3 things you struggle with when it comes to food.

1. Set meal times
2. Healthy choices
3. Getting the balance of foods right
4. Preparation time
5. Lack of knowledge
6. Expense of healthy food
7. Lack of time for seated meals
8. Anything else you struggle with

- Using the chapter on prioritizing 🔗2 to help you if needed, work out how you can incorporate healthier eating habits into your diet.

Plan to:

- Make small lasting changes to your diet every week

- Swap unhealthy food habits for similar, healthier ones

- Incorporate some 'brain food' into your diet daily

Work towards:

- Healthy eating becoming the norm

- Having three set mealtimes a day

- 'Brain foods' becoming a planned part of your diet each day

- Making healthy eating a priority

LINKED TO ⊘

1. Social Butterfly

2. Sort Your Crazy

EXERCISE YOUR MIND
♪♫♪ BETTER WHEN I'M DANCING – MEGHAN TRAINOR ♪♫♪

"The link between exercise and mood is pretty strong. Usually within five minutes after moderate exercise you get a mood-enhancement effect."
-MICHAEL OTTO- PROFESSOR OF PSYCHOLOGY-

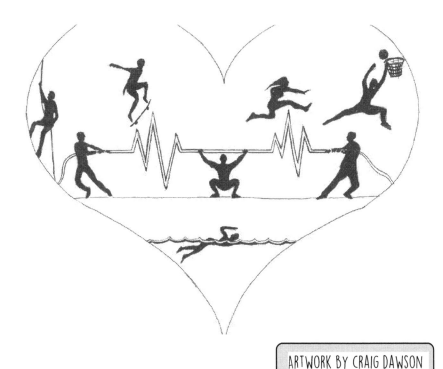

ARTWORK BY CRAIG DAWSON

You had to know I was going to bring this up! Don't you dare skip this chapter, either. Just because you hate exercise doesn't mean it's not important. **Exercise is vital to your mental health**, and I have spent as many years dodging it as a lot of you. But I had good reasons. Kind of. Well, not really. In reality I had excuses, and I used every one in the book.

- I'm tired

- I'm sore

- I have a newborn/toddler/ young child

- I don't have time

- It's too expensive

- Exercise isn't all it's cracked up to be, I'll focus on food.

- I don't have anyone to do it with

- I can't find anything I like doing

- It's raining/hot/windy/ cold

- I'm going tomorrow...

- I don't have the right gear

- They've proven you don't need to exercise to lose weight

That last one was particularly appealing to me. Here was SCIENTIFIC proof that I didn't have to exercise! I mean, how awesome is that! And they're right, to a certain extent. Exercise does not make you thin unless you also eat well.

I once Googled 'does running make you fat,' because I had started running several weeks previously and put ON 2 kgs! The article I read laughingly pointed out that a lot of beginning runners will eat 'naughty' things because they'd 'been for a run,' so it was okay. I thought back to the litre of ice-cream I'd consumed that week and conceded they may be right...

You *will* need to reassess your diet when you start exercising as you're burning more fuel. But make sure you don't use your exercise as an excuse to binge. Have healthy snacks on hand, or better yet, proper meals ready to eat once you come back from exercising. This stops you grabbing the junk and means you can benefit from both the exercise and good food.

But losing weight, however awesome that may be for your self-confidence, is not the best thing about exercising. The best thing is, exercising increases your happiness every single time you do it. And it doesn't matter if you're running, walking, swimming, playing cricket, or mountain biking. It doesn't even matter if you are fit, or a couch potato.

How? Exercise causes endorphins, phenylethylamine, and serotonin to be released. Essentially, happy drugs for your brain. Stress hormones are diminished, your mood brightens, and you are not only more energetic that day, but you sleep better at night, meaning you have an energy knock on into the next day as well!

Exercise, any exercise, will make you happier. Although the powers that be think the best kind for people with mood 'issues' is a 40-minute walk. Apparently, it boosts oxygen levels to the brain...

You see, **your body and mind are connected, and over time exercise causes your brain to re-wire itself in a positive way.** It helps to bounce up your happiness set point, meaning it's easier to be happy every day. Boom! You're cleverer than you thought!

I've come to realize exercise is the most important tool in my good mood arsenal. If I go more than one day without it, I wake up cranky, I find it harder to have positive responses to bad situations (or even neutral ones!), and even the other happiness hacks don't work as well. And I know I'm not the only one.

Many people live stressful lives and need that high-energy exercise for their brains to work on a level keel. It doesn't matter if you're a high-powered professional or a working mum trying to juggle everything, stress causes adrenaline to flood your body, and while that's great for an energy boost in the short term, it has big health and mood ramifications when it is always present.

When we exercise, we metabolize excessive stress hormones — restoring our body and mind to a calmer, more relaxed state. Any form of activity where we "work up a sweat" for five minutes will effectively metabolize off — and prevent the excessive build-up of — stress hormones. Get down and do 50 push-ups, 50 sit-ups, jumping jacks, jump rope, run in place, run up and down the stairs, whatever. By exercising to the point of sweating, we effectively counteract the ill effects of the fight-or-flight response, drawing it to its natural conclusion.[49]

Adrenaline not only keeps us wired, but it can cause strokes, cancer, and high blood pressure if you don't get rid of it. You can say affirmations until the cows come home, but if your system is pumped full of adrenaline, then it's still going to be there when you're done. Exercise is the only way to get it out of your system.

---

[49] http://www.thebodysoulconnection.com/EducationCenter/fight.html

Exercise doesn't have to be boring, or the same thing every day. Think outside the square. If you haven't managed to get out of the house, then run around it! Look on YouTube for a guided workout video. Do crazy dancing with your kids. They'll love it (crazy dancing often ends in breathless giggle fits in our house, which is even better for your mood!). Have a pillow fight with your partner, or a decent roll in the hay. ;-)

My daughter loves GoNoodle. ▶ It's an exercise and meditation program they do at her school, and it's lots of fun. Even dancing to one song in the morning helps lift my spirits (and her attitude). Or download an exercise app to encourage and guide you. The greater range of exercises you introduce, the more motivated and interested you'll be.

Joining an exercise group or class helps with this too. Classes can also add a social element to your life 🔗 1. It can be a bit scary, especially if you're not happy with your body or fitness levels, but I have found it so motivating! And you know what? Nobody's looking at you anyway - they're all worried about themselves!

It doesn't matter if you're new to it - other people will be too. I recently did a couch to 5k running course in my local area. I am not a runner. I didn't even run at school. I have dodgy ankles and knees, amongst other things. But I wanted to be able to run 5 km, so join I did. And I had a blast. All the other people were incredibly friendly. Some were new runners too, and others were getting back into it after time off, and it was such a confidence booster going from strength to strength each week.

I went away for a week in the middle of the course and it was so much harder getting myself out for a run, and keeping a good pace, without other people around. If you don't want to join a group, ask around and find a friend who would be interested in doing a walk with you in the evenings, or when the kids are at school, or any other time that suits. You can kill two birds with one stone and get your exercising and your socializing in one hit.

Start slowly. It is better to do three walks of 15 mins each a week, than to do a 40-minute one once a week. Make sure you listen to your body. No, not while you're sitting on the sofa – get out the door! Focus on your body while exercising. Remember to breathe ✏ 2. Not only does this stop your brain from turning over problems, it helps alert you when you are sore, tired, or need a break.

The idea is to warm your body and breathe more quickly. That's it. That's all you need to do to relieve stress and release those happy chemicals.

You don't need to be exhausted, sweating profusely, or gasping for breath. If you struggle with sore ankles, knees, and hips, etc., then swimming is a great choice. It is one of the most complete forms of exercise anyway, and is easy on your body, as well as great for flexibility. Don't forget to stretch before and after exercise too!

Stretching is just as important, if not more so, than exercising. When you exercise, your tendons and muscles shorten and constrict. Overuse, repetition, and even inactivity all cause hardening, tightening, and inflexibility. This is when injuries happen. Stretching allows your muscles to breath. When the muscles relax, oxygen circulates, waste is removed more effectively, and you let go of tension.

The bestselling book *Stretching to Stay Young* by Jessica Matthews ▶ encourages regular stretching to improve fitness, health, and wellbeing. And bonus, stretching not only helps you move with grace and ease but helps you look younger too. Always warm up before you stretch, not the other way around.

Warming your body raises your muscles temperature for optimum flexibility and helps limit injuries.

Other types of stretching include disciplines such as Yoga and Pilates. These exercises tone your entire body, as well as strengthening your core. They realign things that have moved out of whack over the years and improve flexibility. The gentle (not easy – yoga is way harder than I thought it would be!) exercise helps lower stress, and can be done anywhere, anytime, once you know how.

The trick with exercise is to find something you really enjoy. The more enjoyable the exercise, the more likely you will be to stick to it. I recently started roller derby (yes, like 'Whip It'), and the training sessions run for 2 hours! But I'm having so much fun I don't even notice I'm doing exercise. And it certainly doesn't feel like 2 hours (until the next day anyway).

⊛ Regular aerobic exercise will bring remarkable changes to your body, your metabolism, your heart, and your spirits. It has a unique capacity to exhilarate and relax, to provide stimulation and calm, to counter depression and dissipate stress. It's a common experience among endurance athletes and has been verified in clinical trials that have successfully used exercise to treat anxiety disorders and clinical depression.[50]

If you can't find an exercise you enjoy, then find something that is easy for you to participate in. Live near a pool? Go swimming. Live near the mountains? Go for nature walks. Live in the city? Use bike paths and running trails or do a few laps around the block. A rebounder (mini trampoline) is great if

---

[50] https://www.health.harvard.edu/staying-healthy/exercising-to-relax

you're trapped indoors, as are online instructionals, and they can be made as easy or as hard as you like. Go to a gym or sign up for fitness classes. It doesn't matter. As long as you move your body and energize your mind.

But wait, there's more! Exercise can also lift your mood by giving you a sense of achievement. You got out and did something today. You beat last week's run time. You did an extra lap. Go you! Even if you start off hating exercise, the more you do it the easier it will become, and the more it will energize or relax you, rather than exhausting you. You'll begin to crave it and miss it when you don't do it.

And of course, there's that added bonus of weight loss, when paired with healthy eating. ✪ 3 For some this provides an added boost to their self-esteem, with a knock-on effect of (you guessed it) happiness. But weight loss should not be the main reason for exercising. Exercise should predominately be about your health. Both body, and mind.

Whatever you do, don't wait to become motivated before you start. It won't happen. Motivation, according to Carmen Isaias[52], is a bit of a myth. And I have to agree with her. She says:

"Every goal is more important than the need for motivation to accomplish it. Waiting around for motivation to hit can ironically be the reason we don't do things".
— CARMEN ISAIAS —

---

[52] http://www.huffingtonpost.com/carmen-isais/the-myth-of-motivation_b_8261560.html

Instead of waiting until you're motivated to exercise, set a goal 🔗 4 and then no matter how you're feeling, start. Quite often once you're 10 minutes into it (complaining all the way), you'll realise you are now enjoying it, or at the very least be inspired to continue. Check out the book *Mini Habits* by Stephen Guise▶. He talks about how he built an exercise regime from just one push-up a day.

Be mentally and physically prepared to exercise. Tell yourself you're going to get up and go for a run in the morning. Get all your running gear out and ready. Wake up and say, "I'm going for a run." All these things help prepare you mentally, as well as streamlining the process and making it easy. Exercise, like most things in life, is all about attitude. As soon as you make an excuse, it's all over.

Use exercise in conjunction with other health hacks like eating nutritiously, drinking more water, and catching up on sleep 🔗 5. Notice which healthy actions lift your mood and do more of them! Remember: when you least feel like moving is when you should move the most. Your body (and your brain) desperately need it.

* * *

RECAP 📌

- Exercise is vital to your mental health. It increases your happiness every single time you do it by releasing endorphins and serotonin into your system. Stress hormones are diminished, your mood brightens, and you sleep better at night.

- Exercise is also the only way to get adrenaline out of your system. Adrenaline keeps you wired, and can cause strokes, cancer, and high blood pressure.

- Weight loss should not be the main reason for exercising. Exercise does not make you thin unless you also eat well. Exercise should be about your health. Both body and mind.

- The greater range of exercises you introduce, and the more fun you have doing them, the more motivated and likely to continue exercising you'll be.

- Start slowly. It is better to do three walks of 15 minutes each a week, than to do a 40 minute one once a week. The idea is to warm your body and breathe more quickly. You don't have to be exhausted, sweating, or gasping for breath.

- If you can't find something you enjoy, find something that is close to home and easy to participate in. And don't wait around to become motivated. It'll never happen.

ACTION STEPS ✏

Do now:

- Write a list of all the different exercises you really enjoy, or that you could easily participate in.

- Brainstorm ways of fitting small amounts of exercise into your everyday life.

Plan to:

- Be more active today. Get off the bus a stop early, use the stairs, turn off the TV, go for a walk. Anything that gets you moving.

- Exercise every day. Try new forms of exercise such as dance, roller skating, skiing and see what you enjoy. You might find something you absolutely love, which you may never have considered before.

Work towards:

- Building exercise into your daily routine so it becomes a habit.

- Building up your daily exercise amount to a minimum of 30 minutes a day.

⌾ LINKED TO

1. Social Butterfly

2. Breath and Pose

3. Eat the Food

4. Aim for the Stars

5. Successful Slumber

CREATE A SONG AND DANCE

♪♫♪ BLAME IT ON THE BOOGIE — THE JACKSON 5 ♪♫♪

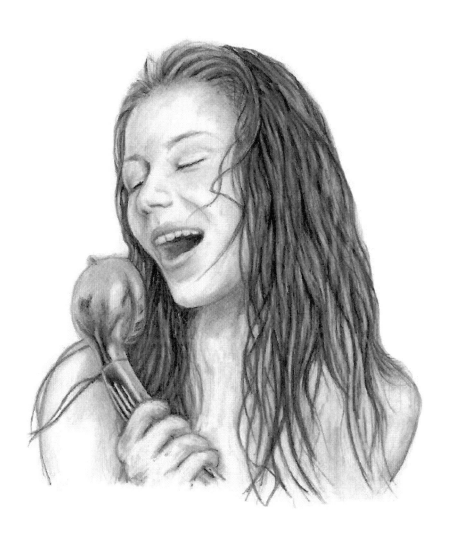

ARTWORK BY CRAIG DAWSON

I was originally going to have the first few lines of 'Blame it on the Boogie' written here so you could sing along, but it turns out the Copyright Act frowns upon things like that. So instead, take this opportunity to look it up on YouTube, iTunes, or Spotify, and crank up the volume. Then back to the book...

Are you still singing? Did you do a little groove? **A good tune is infectious and can set the tone for the next hour or more of your day,** and it is one of the easiest things to implement. Switch on the radio, put on a CD, plug in your phone or iPod. It's really that easy. Music makes us smile ⊘ 1, increases our heart rate, makes us move, and generally enhances our perception of the world.

Humans have used music throughout history, from drums and horns, to fiddles and pipes, to guitars, pianos, and saxophones. Music has always been a part of our lives. And it has evolved right along with humanity. And music, from the dawn of time, has always been used to take its listeners on a journey. Music can make you feel loss and grief, vitality and health, happiness and laughter, or anger and rage. It is incredibly powerful.

> *"Music probably does something unique. It stimulates the brain in a very powerful way, because of our emotional connection with it."*
> -NEUROPSYCHOLOGIST CATHERINE LOVEDAY OF THE UNIVERSITY OF WESTMINSTER-.53

---

53 https://www.theguardian.com/education/2016/oct/24/want-to-train-your-brain-forget-apps-learn-a-musical-instrument

There's a reason why the score to a movie or stage show can make or break it. Music has the ability to compel. It can move us emotionally. A great piece of music can make us cry, laugh, or hide under the bed. When watching a scary scene in a movie people generally do one of two things.

They either cover their eyes, or their ears. Music literally talks to us on an emotional level.

But how many of us really think about what we are listening to? Music is all around us, in elevators and waiting rooms, blaring out in stores and played by buskers in the streets. Our phones are now radios and stereos, and portable speakers let us take our music with us and play it anywhere - loudly!

So how does music affect YOU? Well, everyone is different, but there have been numerous studies done on people, plants and animals, and these are the results.

Cows produced 0.73 litres more milk, per cow, per day when they were exposed to slow music rather than fast music. Scientists hypothesized that the slow music relaxed the cows and reduced their stress levels, leading to an increase in milk. Stress can inhibit the release of oxytocin — a hormone key to the milk-releasing process. [54]

Music such as Aretha Franklin and Beethoven at under 100 beats per minute were the best. Music is the oldest method of relaxation 2 in the world! Your resting heart rate is 60-100 beats a minute so if you're looking for 'restful' music, look under 100 beats a minute, relax, grab some mellow (not mournful) tunes, and put your feet up.

Music actually consists of sound waves that travel through the air at varying frequencies and is then recognized as sound and

[54] http://news.bbc.co.uk/2/hi/science/nature/1408434.stm

music when it reaches our eardrums. So how do plants with no ears (that we know of), grow better with music? Scientists hypothesize that the pressure from sound waves create vibrations that can be picked up by the plants. Several studies also show that not only did seeds germinate faster with music, they grew more leaves, were of greater size, and had other improved characteristics.[55] How crazy is that! The power of music.

And what about people? Well, the studies are conclusive. Music affects us deeply, and it does so from a very young age. Babies as young as 5 months react to happy music and by 9 months are influenced by sad songs.[56] Babies understand emotion before language, so to them, music is just another vehicle to communicate with. And adults are no different, we've just forgotten how intrinsically music speaks to us.

Carol Krumhansl of Cornell University demonstrated that music directly elicits a range of emotions. Happy music is usually in a major key and has a fast tempo. Sad music tends to be played in minor keys and at a slow tempo. Music with a slow tempo can cause your pulse to slow, and your blood pressure to rise, whereas happy music increases your rate of breathing - a physical sign of happiness. Researchers have also discovered that listening to music stimulates many areas in the brain, just like language, and that playing music helps grow areas of your brain, and get it firing. [57]

Music has been proven to lower stress, increase your immune system, and decrease blood pressure. A new study has also found that teaching healthy elderly people to

---

[55] https://dengarden.com/gardening/the-effect-of-music-on-plant-growth
[56] https://medicalxpress.com/news/2008-10-babies-distinguish-happy-sad-music.html
[57] http://cogweb.ucla.edu/ep/Music_Leutwyler_01.html

play music decreases their anxiety, depression, and loneliness. That's pretty cool! [58]

While there's not much research on using music as therapy, four out of five trials that have been undertaken showed music therapy worked better at easing depression symptoms than therapies that did not employ music. It's great for young people who aren't interested in completing talk therapy, and also has a lower dropout rate than traditional therapies.

> ☻ Music recruits neural systems of reward and emotion similar to those known to respond specifically to things such as food, sex, and drugs. The ability of music to produce such intense pleasure, and its stimulation of our body's reward systems, suggests that while music is not necessary for our survival it may be of significant benefit to our mental and physical well-being. [59]

So, what is the best music for a happier mood? It's entirely subjective. Everyone knows what kind of music they enjoy. And like most things in life, what one person loves, another may hate. Here are some tips though.

'Happy' music is generally upbeat (think pop), sad music is often slower and accompanied by sad lyrics (think country). Classical music is often relaxing, although it puts me on edge, so again - subjective.

There don't seem to be any studies (so far) comparing the effects of different genres on various emotions, so instead do your own research. What songs make you feel happier? Which

---

[58] http://www.nytimes.com/1999/06/15/health/vital-signs-therapies-a-fountain-of-youth-in-music-class.html?n
[59] http://www.zlab.mcgill.ca/docs/Blood_and_Zatorre_2001.pdf

songs make you want to dance and move? What songs make you sad and depressed?

From the 1940's until now, our most popular songs on the top 100 have had beats between 117 and 122 a minute. And 120 bpm keeps coming up, study after study, as the tempo that most people feel happier with, which incidentally, is about the same beat as your heart when you're doing physical activity. So, use that as another guide.

For me, pop, rock, and upbeat country all make me happy. Things like techno and house that have a consistent beat can always get me up and dancing, which in turn makes me happy, and ballads, and general 'sad' songs get me down even if I really like the song. Loud rock can be great at de-stressing and shouting along with it can be very therapeutic. But make sure it is energizing you and not making you cranky.

I have to be careful with genres like country and the blues because some songs are happy whereas others are quite melancholy. And I don't really enjoy rap, jazz, or R+B unless they have a really good base melody because they seem too disjointed. But that's me. You will see things very differently.

And if you know the words to the songs, sing along! Hell, even if you don't know the words sing along! See, even when a tune we love is playing, it is still easy for our minds to keep worrying and poking, and prodding, and push the music that's supposed to be helping us, into the background.

When we sing, we are focused on the words, and invested in the music so much that it is almost impossible to ruminate ◎ 3. Oh, happy days! ♪♫♪

When I asked people which song always made them smile, this was their response.

- Katy Perry - 'Roar'
- Nina Simone – 'Feeling Good'
- Tiesto Remix – 'Dancing On My Own'
- Madonna – 'Jump'
- Elton John/Tim Rice – 'Hakuna Matata'
- Pharrell Williams – 'Happy'
- Katrina and the Waves – 'I'm Walking on Sunshine'
- Mark Ronson – 'Uptown Funk'
- Rednex – 'Cotton Eyed Joe'
- Jessie J/Nicki Minaj/Ariana Grande – 'Bang Bang'
- Queen – 'We Will Rock You'
- Taylor Swift – 'Shake It Off'
- Suffragette City – 'Like a Rolling Stone'
- Israel Kamakawiwo'ole – 'Somewhere Over the Rainbow'
- Kenny Loggins - Footloose
- Huey Lewis – 'Power of Love'
- Brad Paisley – 'Today'
- Van Halen – 'Dreams'
- Village People – 'Can't Stop the Music'
- Superchick – 'Get Up'
- Patea Maori Club – 'Poi E'
- Neon Trees – 'Everybody Talks'

- Kacey Musgraves – 'Follow Your Arrow'

- Jessie J – 'It's My Party'

- Phil Lynott – 'Rosalie'

- Tim McGraw – 'Always be Humble and Kind'

- Ed Sheeran – 'Shape of You'

- Sia – 'Alive'

As you can see it's a pretty eclectic mix! Some of these songs would definitely lift my mood whereas others would make it worse, even though I like them. Work out what song makes you happy and go with it.

If you have access to a digital music service like Spotify, you can set up playlists with happiness specifically in mind. That way you can just click play and know the songs are going to lift your mood instead of get you down. So, look for music that has a beat of around 120, as well as music you enjoy, and you should be good to go. Add in a jive and a twist and sing along and you'll be feeling noticeably better, even if you only play one song.

Follow the *Choosing Happy* Playlists on Spotify▶ for a premade selection of feel-good songs in assorted genres. Want to add your favourite song to our playlist? Suggest a song by using the hashtag #choosinghappyplaylist on Instagram, Twitter, or Facebook.

Music is also linked intrinsically with dancing. You hear a favourite song and your feet start to tap. Your shoulders move, your head bobs, and before you know it you're up and dancing! And right there you have a double whammy of happiness. Not only is the music thrumming through your veins and causing joy, but dancing is increasing your pulse, boosting your serotonin levels, and putting you in tune with your body

Studies show dancing is the single best way to immediately boost your happiness. And you don't have to wait to be invited out to a party, or until you hit the club. You can dance whenever you want. Set your alarm to ring in the morning with your favourite tune and get out of bed dancing. Slap on your headphones and have a little bop on the train. Wait for your kids to get home from school and do crazy dancing with them.

It doesn't have to be long or elaborate. Just dance for the space of *one* song, an upbeat song that you love, and I guarantee it will lift your mood.

* * *

RECAP 📌

- Music makes us smile, increases our heart rate, makes us move, and generally enhances our perception of the world. A good tune is infectious and can set the tone for the next hour or more of your day.

- Music from the dawn of time has been used to take us on a journey. It is powerful, and the oldest method of relaxation in the world.

- Researchers have discovered listening to music stimulates many areas of the brain, and that playing music helps get it firing. Happy music is usually in a major key and has a fast tempo.

- Music therapy worked better at easing depression symptoms than therapies that did not employ music. It also has a lower dropout rate than traditional therapies.

- When we sing, we are focused on the words and invested in the music so much it's almost impossible to ruminate.

- Studies show dancing is the single best way to boost your immediate happiness.

ACTION STEPS ✎

Do now:

- Write a list of all the songs that make you feel happy. Ask your friends on Facebook what their favourites are and share yours with them.

- Put on a song you love and dance to it. Right now!

- Look up heidifarrelly on Spotify and start following the *Choosing Happy* playlists. They have happy music by genre. And if you want to swipe the tunes, you can add them straight from the *Choosing Happy* list to your own.

Plan to:

- Work dancing, singing, and listening to music that makes you happy into your everyday life.

- Load your favourite 'happy' songs onto an iPod (or similar) so you can always get a music boost, no matter what you're doing, or where you are.

- Try new music every so often. Not only does this stop you getting bored, but you can discover some amazing songs you would never have found otherwise.

Work towards:

- Dancing to at least one 'happy' song every day.

- Using music to uplift you when you're feeling down, anxious, or stressed.

- Knowing your music. I enjoy country, but I've learnt that when I'm feeling down it's not a great time to listen to it. Listen to your body and mind and learn to pick your music to suit how you're feeling.

LINKED TO

1. Smile – Your Face Won't Crack

2. Relaxation is a Real Thing

3. Thinking Too Much About Crap You Shouldn't

THE WEIRD AND THE WONDERFUL
♪♫♪ BRAVE – SARA BAREILLES ♪♫♪

"There must be something to acupuncture – you never see any sick porcupines."
- BOB GODDARD -

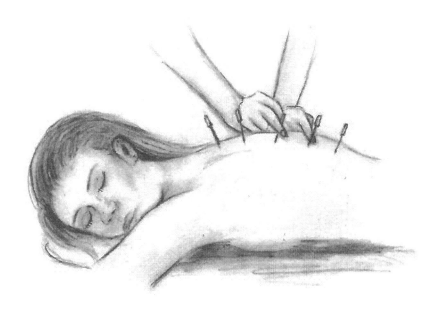

ARTWORK BY CRAIG DAWSON

There are many different therapies that can help with low mood and feelings of sadness. These therapies are not for everyone, and many would consider them 'hokey' or 'wishy washy.' And yet a great deal of people have had a lot of success with the therapies I discuss below, and I do wonder if their level of success correlates with their openness towards the therapy.

Lana Penrose, bestselling author of *The Happiness Quest,*▶ writes about her two-year journey trying everything on offer in her quest for happiness. It was incredibly funny hearing her accounts of visiting a shaman, amongst other things, but even she was surprised by how much some of the alternative therapies helped her.

Each of the following therapies has been demonstrated to improve mood in significant numbers of people. They can help bring about brain change without dulling emotions and have none of the side effects that medication can have ⊘ 1.

Make sure you find a certified practitioner. As with all things, there are people who have spent years perfecting their craft, and others who are just in it for a quick buck. Word of mouth is the best way to find a great practitioner, it ensures that the person you see has good results, not just good marketing!

Try to go into any session with an open mind. After all, as in anything, you only get out what you put in. `If you don't participate, of course it won't work. Nothing will. **Treatment is not something done *to* us. *We* are the only ones that have direct access to our minds and emotions, and as such *we* have control over our treatment.** Give them an honest go.

I've briefly outlined each of the therapies to give you a basic understanding of them and have provided further reading links if you are interested in knowing more.

Kinesiology

Kinesiology▶ does not treat or diagnose diseases. It is more concerned with balancing the body's energies. It involves muscle testing to determine what's going on inside your mind and body, incorporates positive ideas and affirmations, and attempts to realign your chakras, and boost your chi. Kinesiology works on the premise that there is energy flowing through your body that relates to every muscle, tissue, and organ.

Kinesiology bypasses conscious thinking, and instead uses muscle testing to help identify, fix, and balance blockages in the energy flow. It allows you to take charge of how you relate to the past, present, and future, and helps you access the movement of energy around the body and brain. In other words, it lets your body do the talking!

It's great for people who don't necessarily want to talk about their problems, as it taps into the body for answers instead. You'll be asked to provide detailed information about your medical history and what you want out of the session, but you don't discuss your emotions.

Kinesiology can boost mood by helping you overcome past traumas, eliminating stress, releasing fears, and identifying nutritional deficiencies. It uses a range of different methods to balance your bodies energies. These include tracing or massaging meridians, light and colour frequency, tapping, breath work and physical releases, belief system reframing, relaxation and visualisation work, homeopathic remedies, and nutrition.

Animal Assisted Therapy (AAT) or Pet Assisted Therapy (PAT), Animal Assisted Activities (AAA), and Pets

Pet therapy▶ is any guided interaction between people and trained animals. Dogs and cats are the most widely used for AAT, PAT, and AAA, but horses, guinea pigs, and other animals can also be used. Animals are the best listeners and don't judge you on anything they hear either! They can sense your feelings, and can help decrease your feelings of loneliness, isolation, and anxiety, and in doing so lift your mood, and your outlook on life.

While pet therapy is used more for people with serious physical and mental problems, it can also be helpful for those of us suffering low mood or anxiety.

AAT is undertaken by a trained handler and you are fitted to your ideal animal, which is pretty cool. It is essentially the planned inclusion of an animal into your life for treatment purposes. Some things to consider would be allergies or fears of specific animals.

PAT is slightly different in that it uses animals in recreation and visitation programs which aren't as specific, such as horseback riding or nursing home visits. They can also hold duties such as seizure dogs and seeing eye dogs.

While owning a pet is not considered AAT, **research has long shown that pets have a positive therapeutic effect on vulnerable people, and doctors, therapists, and other health professionals all agree animals are great antidotes to loneliness.**

Being responsible for the care of a pet can give us something else to focus on. Someone outside of ourselves needs us, relies on us, and gives us purpose. Pets give us a daily routine to follow, and the fate of our pets can anchor us to life at times when we don't want to participate. They save countless lives just by being there and loving you unconditionally. That kind of companionship should never be underestimated.

> (☻) Stroking, hugging, or otherwise touching a loving animal can rapidly calm and soothe us when we're stressed or anxious. The companionship of a pet can also ease loneliness, and most dogs are a great stimulus for healthy exercise, which can substantially boost your mood and ease depression.[60]

Whether you participate in AAT, PAT, AAA, or simply own a pet, being able to stroke or groom an animal is incredible soothing, and they can have an extraordinary calming effect. Each of these are tools that can be used by themselves or with other therapies to achieve goals, calm the mind, and help overcome sadness and loneliness.

Five Elements acupuncture

Five Elements acupuncture ▶ is an ancient form of acupuncture that has been around for thousands of years. The Chinese used it to specifically focus on an individual's emotional wellbeing instead of their physical wellbeing. It provides people with a capacity to process things and break through emotional blockages to let anger and sadness flow naturally.

Five Elements acupuncture is based on the foundation that each one of us have one element that is both a strength and a weakness in our lives, and this creates an imbalance. It aims to correct that imbalance so your whole body can heal and move

---

[60] https://www.helpguide.org/articles/mental-health/mood-boosting-power-of-dogs.htm

forward. The fire element is associated with joy, earth with sympathy, wood with anger, metal with grief, and water with fear. They are like parts of our personality.

Five Elements works by positively affecting the quality of your body's energy or 'chi.' If you think of your energy as a river, and your emotional blockages as dams or partial blockages in that river, you will begin to see what a big difference it can make. During each session, your practitioner will assess your blockages between the meridian points, and then pick specific acupuncture points for that day.

You will probably need around 4 treatments, perhaps more depending on the severity of your problem, and each session will last 45 minutes to an hour. Unlike in traditional acupuncture, the needles are not usually left in but inserted and then removed immediately.

Art Therapy and Arts Therapies

Yup, it's subtle, but they are different! Art therapy ▶ uses the visual arts such as drawing, painting, and sculpture to improve your physical, mental, and emotional well-being, to assist people in times of emotional distress, and encourage learning, self-reflection, and expression. Arts therapists ▶ on the other hand, use dance/movement and drama as well as visual art making to achieve the same results.

Now I don't know about you, but I don't have an artistic bone in my body. Well, I craft, but when it comes to drawing and painting I'm terrible! But that's okay because you don't have to have any kind of artistic flair to participate in art therapy. And you don't have to be a dancer or an actor to participate in arts therapies either. The emphasis is not on the end product of your work, but on the process of creating and reflecting on meaning.

Every human being has imagination and creativity, and art therapy is all about tapping into those traits. Art therapists are highly trained and work with their clients to help them reflect on their own work, discover meanings in it, and empower them. It can help participants who find it hard to express themselves verbally share their fears and thoughts in a safe environment and identify concerns.

> *Art that has depth has a strong impact on the spirit, emotion, mood, and thoughts of a human being.*
> -LI SHAN-

Art therapy has seen proven results in patients suffering from a range of disorders and health conditions. These include depression, anxiety, distress, low self-esteem, anger, confusion, coping skills, some physical and mental components of Alzheimer's, reduction in PTSD symptoms, and quality of life and general health also improves[61]. I mean, wow.

Unfortunately, while art therapy and arts therapies have been recognised and regulated worldwide, they are generally not offered free to the people who need it the most. Which means it will hit your back pocket. My closest art therapy group offers sessions for $50, which means a 6-week stint would set you back $300! If money's not an issue then I urge you to give it a go, but if it is then consider doing art in your own home without the added expense.

Just like affirmations and gratitude journals have been found to improve mood when done on a daily basis, so has doing creative pursuits. For you, this may be drawing or sculpting.

---

[61] https://www.ncbi.nlm.nih.gov/books/NBK279641/

You might make jewellery or paint. Whatever it is, use it as a release. A chance to express yourself without words, get your feelings and thoughts out of your brain and into a different form of expression.

Emotional Freedom Technique (EFT), or 'Tapping'

EFT is a form of psychological acupressure and is based on the same meridians and pressure points as traditional acupuncture. The idea that electromagnetic energy passes through our body and can affect our health (what EFT is based on), is only beginning to be understood in Western cultures, but it has a very high rate of success, and knowledge about it is spreading rapidly.

EFT is very easy to learn and can be done anywhere, which is the biggest difference between it and traditional acupuncture. Once you have learned where and how it is performed, you can combine tapping with positive affirmations ✍ 2 to "short-circuit" an emotional block, helping to balance the mind and the body.

There are many guided EFT videos on YouTube ▶ that will help you learn general techniques, and more specific ones. There is also a great article on tapping at Mercola.com[62] that will have you underway in no time, but here's some tips to help you get started.

- Tapping is performed using the fingertips (not the pads) as they have their own meridian points.

- You will tap in specific locations but don't worry if you're not in the exact spot - it will still help.

- Tap solidly but not hard enough to hurt yourself.

---

[62] http://eft.mercola.com/

- Remove jewellery, watches, and glasses as they can interfere with the electromagnetic pulse.

- You can perform EFT with the index and middle fingers on one hand as is traditional, or all fingers on both hands. I find this easier.

- Tapping starts at the top of your head and continues down your body in order, making it easy to remember. There are 10 different points.

- Once you know your meridian points and have chosen an affirmation you can begin. It will only take about a minute each round.

- Tune in to the problem you are having, or trying to solve, and hold it in your mind.

- As you begin tapping, start saying your affirmations in a loud, positive way.

- Continue your affirmations as you complete the round of tapping.

You can do tapping when you wake up as part of your morning routine, before meals, when you go to the bathroom, when you're stopped at traffic lights, or any other time throughout the day. Try it out before you disregard it entirely. You might be surprised! I find tapping helps me break away from negative thoughts and focus my mind on the process of tapping itself. That, for me, is a big win, even if there are no other effects.

I have even used tapping in the middle of the night as a diversion to get myself back to sleep before my busy brain takes over ⊘ 3. Beats counting sheep any day!

There are many other types of alternative therapies, but these are the ones that have proven the most helpful to a broad range of people. I guess the bottom line with any alternative therapy is this: While some of them have thousands of years' history, many have little to no scientific evidence that they work. However, we also used to think the world was flat - until we knew that it wasn't.

Some people put the positive change in mood after alternative therapies down to a placebo effect. Essentially - you think you're going to get better, so you do. While this is possible (although highly improbable due to the years they have been around, and the number of people the therapies have helped), it doesn't really matter whether it is or not. If it makes you feel better, that's awesome!

So, take the therapies as you find them. If they work for you, great. If they don't, try another one, or one of the many hacks in this book. You are only limited by what you choose to try.

* * *

RECAP 🔖

- There are many different therapies that can help with low mood and sadness. They can help bring about brain change without dulling emotions and have none of the side effects that medication can have.

- Try to go into any session with an open mind. Treatment is not something done to us. We are the only ones that have direct access to our minds and emotions, and as such we have control over our treatment.

- Kinesiology is concerned with balancing the body's energies. It uses muscle testing to help identify, fix, and balance blockages in the energy flow. It's great for people who don't want to talk about their problems as it taps into the body for answers instead.

- Being able to stroke or groom an animal is incredibly soothing, and they can have an extraordinary calming effect. Animals are the best listeners and can help decrease your feelings of loneliness, isolation, and anxiety, and in doing so lift your mood, and your outlook on life.

- Five Elements acupuncture provides people with a capacity to process things, and break through emotional blockages to let anger and sadness flow naturally. Unlike in traditional acupuncture, the needles are inserted and then removed immediately.

- Art therapy uses visual arts such as drawing, painting and sculpture to improve your physical, mental and emotional well-being. Art therapists use dance, movement and drama to achieve the same results. The emphasis is not on the end product, but on the creative process and reflecting on meaning.

- EFT is a form of psychological acupressure and is based on the same meridians and pressure points as traditional acupuncture. It is easy to learn and can be done anywhere to relieve stress and anxiety and break away from negative thoughts.

ACTION STEPS ✎

Do now:

- Pick one alternative therapy you would be willing to try and start looking for a practitioner.

- Give tapping a try. It will literally take you 5 minutes to learn and try.

Plan to:

- Try at least one alternative therapy. Commit to it wholeheartedly and track your progress. Go into it knowing what you would see as a success. Often, we set a goal and then move it when we get close to it or surpass it. Writing down our expectations and starting points helps us to see whether something is working or not. 🌀 4

Work towards:

- Trying each of these alternative therapies and anything else that you think may help. What have you got to lose? Except money. Damn it, there's always a down side! Don't send yourself broke trying everything - that's not going to help your mood! Instead, look for therapies that may be offered free or discounted through your health insurance, local area, or a friend.

LINKED TO 🌀

1. Give Me the Drugs

2. Say it Like You Mean it

3. Successful Slumber

4. Aim for the Stars

GIVE ME THE DRUGS
♪♫♪ I FEEL GOOD — JAMES BROWN ♪♫♪

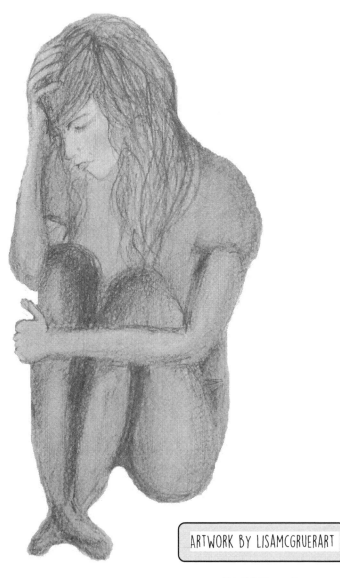

ARTWORK BY LISAMCGRUERART

I wanted to talk to you briefly about medication. Not anti-depressants specifically because this isn't a depression book, but medication in general. I feel it's something I need to touch on as it's an important but not often spoken of subject.

Way back at the beginning of this book we talked about low mood being like a headache. Headaches can be debilitating - especially if they are frequent. And yet they are something everyone feels comfortable talking about and are happy to take medication for. So why, when it comes to your mental health, something that has an impact on our entire lives, do we get all squirrely?

People think I should be able to handle my illnesses without medicine. In reality, without medicine, my illnesses would handle me.
-SARAH CEASAR-

Not only would most sufferers never consider taking medication for mood until they were forced to, but the general populace would be a little bit askance if you did decide to take it. Because you should totally just be able to pull your head in, carry on, and stop being so soft, right?

Wrong. That's not the way mental health works. **Just like you often need help to get rid of a headache, so too may you need a bit of extra help getting your mood back on track.** And I'm not just talking about anti-depressants, although they are an important part in many people's journey. I'm talking about any health issues that may be negatively impacting your mental health and their medication. Here's an example.

I've been struggling for a while. Different from my depression in that I could be happy, but similar in the fact that I was exhausted and struggling emotionally. Which I've found really hard because I had been doing so well! But 6 months ago, I really hit a wall and I went to the doctor in tears. I was dizzy and nauseated, exhausted and emotional, and skipping periods.

After lots of blood tests (because I hadn't had enough during IVF...) I finally got an answer. It wasn't a great answer, but at least I could start making sense of everything. Turns out I have Premature Ovarian Failure (POF). Essentially, I was going into menopause at 35. Which explained a lot! The previous infertility, the tiredness, the crankiness, and a host of other symptoms.

I saw a fabulous specialist and she explained what I could do to combat the symptoms. I had to start Hormone Replacement Therapy (HRT) because I was far too young to be going without oestrogen. My oestrogen was so low the test results read 'nil detected.' My friend (also a doctor) suggested I frame it as she's never seen a reading that low! Lack of oestrogen has all sorts of side effects. Essentially everything I'd been feeling plus osteoporosis down the track and other fun things...

But HRT! Wasn't that super bad stuff that has all kinds of side effects? The specialist explained that it had a worse rap than it should, and that tests were actually really positive for people my age. And if I didn't take it I'd have osteoporosis and be breaking bones by 50. Some choice!

I was feeling so crap by then I didn't really care anyway. I practically screamed 'give me the drugs!' Which in hindsight was a sign of how bad I was feeling as I've never taken anything more exciting than Nurofen - except in childbirth. After a bone scan I filled my script and started on what would be a daily pill for the next 15-20 years.

And it was the best thing I've ever done. It's been three months, and I feel so much better already! I'm sleeping through the night again. I don't have to pick which things I do in a day because I'm not exhausted part way through. My emotions ⌀ 1 are far more level and I can start exercising ⌀ 2 again (no more dizziness), which in turn has boosted my mood.

Why have I told you this (long winded) story? Because it doesn't matter how many changes you implement in your life, **if you're not well or if you are lacking something physically, you cannot be whole mentally.** And that's what I want to emphasize. Medication is there for a reason. If you have a serious physical or mental health issue, then you should take the drugs. Just like a headache, remember?

If you've seen a doctor and they've recommended something that will help, and the only reason you're not doing it is because you don't want to be 'that person' who needs a pill to be happy, then pull your head out of your arse! How lucky are you that there is something that can help! So many people have undiagnosed problems, or they have things like endometriosis or MS which have no cure and can only be managed. Take the pill, feel better, and then under your doctor's guidance work on implementing other strategies that will help.

You may only need the medication for a short while, or like me you may need it for the foreseeable future, but if it makes you well and happy then it doesn't matter. What matters is that you do everything in your power to live a life that is extraordinary. And sometimes that means shouting 'give me the drugs!'

It's always worth getting a second opinion or seeing a specialist doctor when making big changes. Even excellent doctors are wrong sometimes or simply don't know what the best solution for you is. Do your own research (always using reputable sources as there's a lot of misinformation out there), find a doctor you trust, or talk to a few and see what they come up with.

I saw a specialist because both GP's I saw said they couldn't prescribe anything 'til I got worse. Did I mention the 'nil detected' oestrogen? Yeah. Not cool. You know yourself better than anyone else, regardless of the degree they hold. Keep pushing if you think you need to. I'm so glad I did.

> ☢ "We can make medications part of the solution rather than the problem by having meaningful discussions with consumers about medications before they are prescribed (and addressing any underlying concerns)." [63]

Sometimes medication is not the answer though. Unfortunately, there seems to be a lot of over-prescription happening around the globe for almost every physical and mental condition. A friend of mine

---

[63]https://nswmentalhealthcommission.com.au/sites/default/files/uploa ds/Medication%20and%20mental%20illness%20perspectives%20Nov% 202015.pdf

was prescribed painkillers and anti-depressants for really bad PMS symptoms. Her GP just kept prescribing more and more medication, but nothing was helping. She finally went to a different doctor, who took her off all the medication, and solved her problem in 2 minutes flat.

If you are prescribed medication you don't think you need, that isn't working, or is making you feel worse, then get back to your doctor and start pushing for change or consult a different physician. Medication is there to improve your life, not make it worse.

Medication, when used in the right way, can be a Godsend. So, don't discount anti-depressants or other medication just because it's not the socially accepted thing to do. If medication is the key to helping you stay healthy, both physically and mentally, then that can only be good.

* * *

RECAP 📌

- Just like you often need help getting rid of a headache, so too may you need help getting your mood back on track.

- It doesn't matter how many changes you implement in your life, if you're not well, or if you're lacking something physically, you cannot be whole mentally.

- If medication helps you stay healthy both physically and mentally then that can only be good.

ACTION STEPS ✎

Do now:

- If you suspect everything is not 100% physically then book an appointment with your doctor and get them to do a blood screen. Make sure things like vitamin B12, vitamin D, ferritin, folate, blood glucose, liver, thyroid, and hormones are covered as these are pretty common culprits for zapping your energy and messing with your mood.

Plan to:

- Work with your doctor on assessing your needs and creating an action plan. This could include exercise, healthy eating, and medication if needed.

Work towards:

- Combatting any medical issues so your journey to excellent mental health will be less of a struggle.

LINKED TO ◎

1. Emotional Rollercoaster

2. Exercise Your Mind

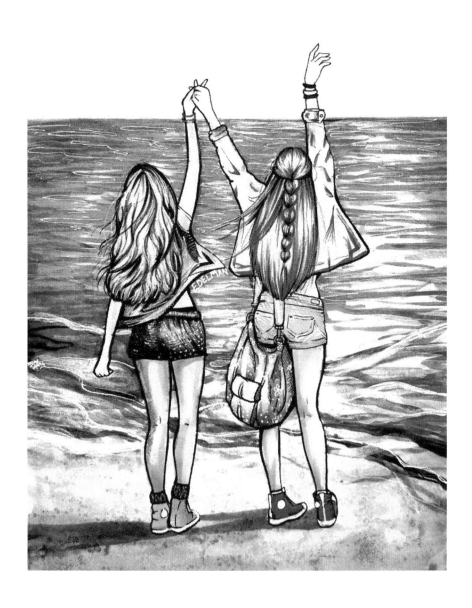

ARTWORK BY KELLY EDELMAN

CONNECT

LEARNING TO INTERACT SOCIALLY, GROW AS A PERSON, AND MAKE MEANINGFUL CONNECTIONS IN YOUR DAY-TO-DAY LIFE CAN BE INCREDIBLY HARD FOR THOSE OF US WITH MOOD ISSUES. BUT IT IS ALSO MASSIVELY IMPORTANT.

CONNECTION IS KEY TO CREATING AND MAINTAIN HEALTHY RELATIONSHIPS, INTERACTING WITH THE WORLD AROUND YOU, FINDING JOY THROUGH GROWTH AND GIVING, AND ULTIMATELY TO OVERCOMING LOW MOOD.

SOCIAL BUTTERFLY
♪♫♪ ROAR – KATY PERRY ♪♫♪

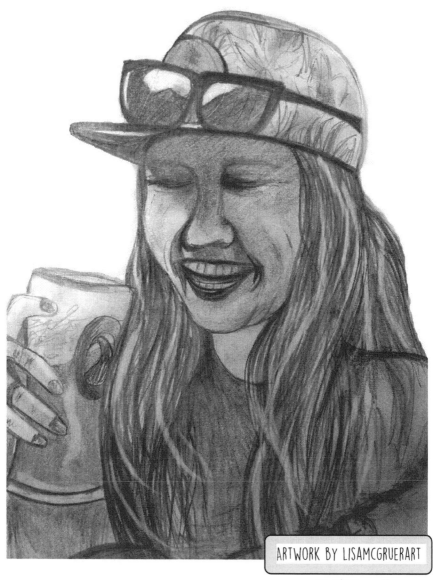

ARTWORK BY LISAMCGRUERART

When you're feeling sad, or down, it's so easy to closet yourself away. To isolate yourself from people and retreat into your own little cocoon of silence. But typically, the more you retreat into yourself, or your four walls, the harder it is to put yourself back out there.

I don't know about you, but I am happy in my own company. Even when I'm well, often the thought of going out and catching up with people is not as enticing as having some 'alone' time. It's easy to tell yourself that you'd rather sit on the sofa watching TV because you're tired either mentally or physically. But the reality is, social interaction can energize and buoy you. And it is now something that I make myself do. I just have to get myself out the door!

If getting out the door is something you struggle with too, consider putting things in place that will help you. Organize a car pool so you will either need to be there for others or they'll be banging on your door! Or try going to social gatherings straight from work. I find this much easier than relaxing at home and then having to go out again!

One of the most important things you can do to lift your mood is to socialize. Human beings as a whole are hardwired for connection. We need that friendship, that closeness with other people. It is an intrinsic part of our makeup. And when we shut ourselves off from all of that, we close the door on one of the most healing and restorative things for our spirit.

Close relationships with family and friends provide us with not only love and support, but increased feelings of self-worth and belonging. If you sit at home, you run the risk of feeling lonely and unloved. And loneliness is a big issue for those struggling with low mood. Not to mention you've given yourself space and time to let all those negative thoughts swirl in your head.

☻ Did you know that we are 30 times more likely to laugh when we are hanging out with friends?[64] This is because laughter is in itself a form of communication, not, as most people believe, a reaction to a joke or media. Science shows that laughter is mostly used to show people we like and understand them. The huge increase in laughter when socializing makes sense when you understand this. And of course, laughter is the same as smiling ✎1. It gives you that instant feeling of happiness. See how important socializing is?

It is actually impossible for your brain to function normally without social contact, and yet you are voluntarily isolating yourself. Get out the door! I know some of you are shy, introverted, or think of yourselves as 'loners,' but you need to make the effort to get out there. I'm not saying it's going to be easy, but I am saying it's going to be worth it in the long run.

Martin Seligman, an American psychologist who is regarded by many as the founder of positive psychology states:

"How do extremely happy people differ from the rest of us? It turns out there's one very surprising way. They're extremely social."
- MARTIN SELIGMAN -

---

[64] http://www.bbc.com/news/health-29754636

Everybody has different social needs, because everyone is different. Wild, right? If you're an introvert your idea of quality socialisation may be a quiet coffee with a close friend. If you're an extrovert, you probably prefer chatting with a group of people. And if you're an introverted extrovert (real thing, people), you probably like a bit of both. And that's fine! It doesn't matter what form your socialization takes. It's just important that you have it in your life on some level.

Shyness, or lack of social skills can be a huge stumbling block for many. And unfortunately, our hyper-culture where everything is instantaneous has made people impatient. We don't want to waste time waiting for shy people to adjust or find their way out of their shells. We want to smash out that socialization like it's just another check on our to-do list. And this means the naturally shy are often left behind.

If you know you struggle socially, encourage your mates to call in, drag you out, or simply stay in with you for a bit. Let them know that just because you don't want to meet all the school mums for coffee doesn't mean you wouldn't mind seeing just them for a catch up.

It's not up to the extroverts in our group of friends to make all the effort though. Forcing yourself into social situations when you're shy isn't enough. You have to be present, and actually make an effort to interact. Sitting in a corner feeling miserable because no-one is talking to you is a problem *you* have the power to solve. Here's some ideas to get you started.

- If you're not social by nature, or you worry about what to talk about in a social setting, make a list of conversation starters or things you've been up to. Nine times out of ten you'll find you don't need them, but if it makes you less anxious – go for it!

- Go out with a few people at once so you don't have to bear as much of the conversation. You can talk very little but still be part of a happy, social gathering.

- Participate in a group activity where you can laugh and have fun – without the stress of having to make conversation.

- Be aware of those around you. Not just the uber social person you're wishing you could be like. Look around. Roughly half of us admit to being shy. Who else can you see that's hanging back? Listening instead of talking? Go say hi! Being there simply isn't enough.

- Employ the 'one' strategy. Pick one person, go up and say hi, and ask them one question or tell them one thing about yourself. Conversations and friendships have started from a lot less.

- Admit you're shy. Sometimes that's all it takes for people to realise they're not the only one struggling, or to make more of an effort to include you.

- What if you don't have any close friends? Or any friends that are close by? Then begin to build new friendships. Your best friend could be a person you haven't even met yet. I love this truth. Building friendships is a great way to combat loneliness.

- Start a conversation with a stranger, ▶ put yourself out there in social gatherings, or join a club doing something that interests you. ⌾ 2 You can use the 'one' strategy for this too. Just focus on one thing at a time. Okay, today I just need to send an inquiry... okay, today I just need to sign up... okay, today I just need to turn up... okay, today I just need to meet one new person. It is a simple way of breaking big things down into more manageable, less terrifying ones.

We need to see socialization as an investment in our lives. The initial outlay may be a sacrifice for where you're at now, it might be a challenge or a little painful at times, but the benefits far outweigh the costs, if you are willing to take the plunge. And not only does socializing mean you'll be meeting new people, and greeting old friends, you will also be building your self-confidence and your self-esteem.

It's the friends we meet along the way that help us appreciate the journey.

When we socialize, we need to think carefully about who we choose to spend time with. In the same way that positive people make you feel uplifted and energized, negative people can leave you feeling more sad, angry, and drained. So, while it's important to help friends when they are down, you need to minimize the time you spend with negative people while you're struggling with sadness yourself.

And just as it's important for us to surround ourselves with positive people, so too is it important for our friends. Make sure you give your friends the best of you. If you go out thinking you're going to have a terrible time, then chances are, you will. Even when you've forced yourself out the door, you can enjoy yourself. Be thankful you have friends that want to hang out. Be grateful 𝒪 3 for their time, their effort, and their inclusion of you in their lives. Enjoy the moment and celebrate the connection.

That's not to say you can't talk to your friends about your problems. I highly encourage you to do so. But be wise about who you share with. Downloading to all and sundry doesn't help, and in fact it can put people off. Choose someone you know and trust and be honest with them. Tell them you're struggling.

You know they will help you, and support you any way they can, and sometimes just sharing what you're going through can help lift your mood. You need strong people around you who are understanding, so talk to them, listen to their answers and really hear what they're saying. Don't immediately dismiss what they say about you, or your situation. Remember, when we are sad our life view is distorted.

Good friends often see us more clearly than we see ourselves. They help you see the positive and work out the negative. If I had talked to my friends sooner, I'm sure I would have addressed my depression and dealt with it a lot earlier than I did. Don't underestimate how much your friends want to help you. They really do. And it took me a long time to learn this. It is never a sign of weakness to ask for or receive help from friends. One day you will be there to help others. And just as your friends supported you, so too can you support them.

If you know a friend is struggling don't give up on them. You don't necessarily have to say anything to make them feel better. Just sitting with someone, offering companionship and solidarity in tough times, can mean more than you think. It demonstrates to your friends that you care about them, and that their friendship is important to you.

Another trick to encouraging positive social interactions is to deliberately talk about something good that is happening in your life, even when you feel like everything is falling apart.

Your friends in turn will probably tell you something good that's happening in theirs.

Positivity begets positivity. Feed off each other's happiness. Let it buoy you. This is what socializing is all about! When you leave, you will not only have talked through a problem with a friend, you will have shared a happiness with them. Both of these things are equally important.

Don't have the time for catch ups? Make the time! Prioritize ⟁ 4 your life and ensure you can socialize even once a week for half an hour. Even just lingering at school drop offs, at the coffee shop, at the proverbial water cooler to chat to people, can help far more than you would have imagined.

Be genuine in your interactions with those around you. Your barista, your neighbour, the checkout girl, and the bus driver. Smile, say thank you. Ask about their day, their shift, or compliment them. Even a 30-second conversation can form part of your social needs, and small interactions can not only have a positive impact on your day, but on others as well.

Stop looking for excuses on why you can't socialize and listen to me carefully. If you do not connect with other people in some way, shape, or form, you will run the risk of never being as happy as you want to be. Socialization is that important!

* * *

RECAP ✄

- One of the most important things you can do to lift your mood is to socialize. Human beings need connection, and close relationships with family and friends not only provide us with love and support, but increased feelings of self-worth and belonging.

- It is actually impossible for your brain to function normally without social contact, and typically the more you retreat into yourself, or your four walls, the harder it is to put yourself back out there.

- Everybody has different social needs. For some it may be having a quiet cuppa with a friend. Others may prefer to chat with a group of people. Everyone is different.

- If you know you struggle socially, encourage your mates to call in, drag you out, or simply stay in with you for a bit. Or employ the 'one' strategy in social situations. Pick one person, go and say hi, and ask them one question or tell them one thing about yourself.

- Build new friendships. Your best friend could be someone you haven't even met yet.

- Don't underestimate how much your friends want to help you. It is never a weakness to ask for or receive help from a friend. They often see us more clearly than we see ourselves.

- In the same way that positive people make you feel uplifted and energized, negative people can leave you feeling more sad, angry and drained.

- If you know a friend is struggling don't give up on them. Just sitting with someone, offering companionship and support can mean more than you think.

- Even a 30-second conversation can form part of your social needs, and small interactions can not only have a positive impact on your day, but on others as well.

ACTION STEPS ✎

Do now:

- Message someone you haven't seen in a while and arrange a catch-up. A real one. Face to face, not screen to screen.

- Write a list of everyone you could catch up with throughout your week.

- Write a list of any groups you would like to join. This could be a gym, a language course, a hiking group, or something as simple as a coffee group.

Plan to:

- Make more time for the people who matter. Chat with a loved one or friend, call your parents, or play with the kids.

- Prioritize socialization. It is not just frivolous, but something incredibly important to our mental wellbeing. Set up a communication tab in your diary and write three names. One to text, one to call, one to catch up with. That's it. If you do more – awesome, but every week make sure you do each of those things.

- Make 3 extra connections today. Wave at a neighbour, learn the name of someone new, stop to chat to someone in a shop.

Work towards:

- Sitting yourself next to someone you don't know at social gatherings. This not only means you build new friendships, it's also great for your confidence.

- Being social on some level at least once a day. Even if it's just having a chat over the fence with your neighbour.

- Hosting a social gathering. Invite good friends, and those you are just getting to know. Talk to everyone, not just those you are closest to. If you find this sort of thing stressful make it easier on yourself by having it at a park, or a coffee shop, or by getting everyone to bring a plate of food to share. This not only takes the pressure off, but it makes people feel more like they are a part of things. Wine and cheese nights are always great fun too.

- Saying 'yes' when people ask you out to coffee, dancing, a movie, or an event. Being more social can really open up your world, if you let it.

LINKED TO

1. Smile- Your Face Won't Crack

2. Learning to Grow

3. Great Attitute

4. Sort Your Crazy

GIVE A LITTLE

♪♫♪ POCKET FULL OF SUNSHINE — NATASHA BEDINGFIELD ♪♫♪

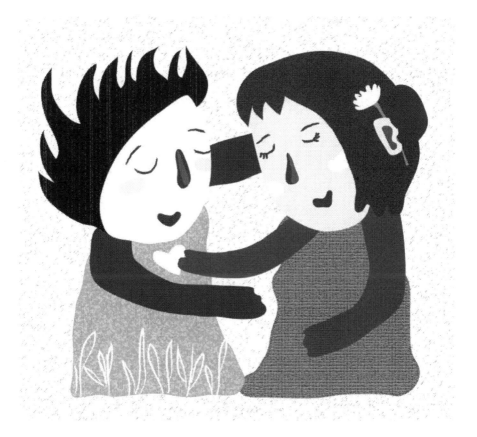

ARTWORK BY MJ.OANNE

When Christmas comes around I'm like a kid in a candy store. Not because I love receiving gifts, but because I love giving them! My sister-in-law is the same. She described it as that excitement and joy of giving something to a loved one, and knowing you nailed it. That they loved your gift and know how much thought went into it.

Giving is powerful! And it doesn't matter what form your giving takes. The outcome is the same. **When you increase the happiness of those around you, you increase your own as a by-product.**

My daughter had a home reader from school when she was six about doing things for others and being kind. It was called *Have You Filled a Bucket Today?* by Carol McCloud▶. They used an analogy of filling an invisible bucket through acts of kindness and giving to others, which in turn fills your bucket at the same time. I thought the analogy was a bit silly at first, but the more I thought about it, the more I realised it was very true! Your actions have a profound effect not only on others, but on yourself.

Giving helps create connections between people, and generally makes the world a better place. When we hear the word 'giving' we automatically think money. But it's not all about cash. We can give of our time, love, and energy. It is said happiness is best achieved 'sideways on,' which means instead of focusing on ourselves, we should focus on the happiness of those around us. So, if you want to feel good, give.

I grew up knowing the 'golden rule' off by heart, as did most of my peers. "Do unto others as you would have them do unto you." And while people are happy to do this in an offhanded way, we don't often put a lot of thought into it. When was the last time you actually stopped and thought, 'What can I do to show someone I care today?' Last week? Last year? It's simply not at the forefront of people's minds. And it should be. Because caring about others is fundamental to our own happiness!

Imagine if everyone in your workplace decided to treat others with the respect, understanding, and love that they would like to receive. The change would be incredible! People would start to enjoy coming to work (a miracle in itself). Colleagues would listen to each other's ideas. People would start to feel a sense of belonging. This would lead to staff working better together, and more cohesion in the business. Staff would know they were valued, and they would work hard to ensure they remained that way.

Putting such a simple concept as the golden rule into action could change an entire workplace into a thriving hub, where people were supported, and valued, and where they put the happiness of others at the front of their mind.

Now imagine if the whole world did that.

The term 'pay it forward' has been around for a long time, but the book by Catherine Ryan Hyde▶, and subsequent movie in 2000, bought it into the public's eye and made it a global phenomenon.

In 2007 Blake Beattie founded the 'Pay It Forward Day',▶ which states, 'Any random act of kindness can cause a positive ripple effect restoring our faith in the love and compassion of the human spirit. There is tremendous power and positive energy in giving. Pay It Forward Day is about all people, from all walks of life, giving to someone else. It is a powerful reminder of the difference we can all make.'

I can't even comprehend how much that would change the society we live in. You don't have to wait for it to become a global movement though. You can start changing the world around you right now, by giving of yourself.

And that's the crazy awesome thing about giving! People you give to are in turn more likely to give to others because of it. It is like a great big circle of happiness and giving. And giving can be done at any age. Even pre-school aged children understand the concept.

☻ Researchers found that "people in general felt happier when they were asked to remember a time they bought something for someone else — even happier than when they remembered buying something for themselves. This happiness boost was the same regardless of whether the gift cost $20 or $100. The happier participants felt about their past generosity, the more likely they were in the present to choose to spend on someone else instead of themselves. According to the authors, the results suggest a kind of "positive feedback loop" between kindness and happiness, so that one encourages the other.[65]

And you can start that! You may never see the ripples that your gift created, but they could continue indefinitely in small ways, from person to person. How's that for a legacy of happiness?

I created little 'UplifTin' cards last year. They were a 3-inch square card that you could write a wee note on, give to people, and keep to look back on when you were low. The premise was simple. Instead of just thinking, 'Gee, she's doing a great job with her health/kids/job,' you could write an encouraging note

[65]https://greatergood.berkeley.edu/article/item/kindness_makes_you_happy_and_happiness_makes_you_kind

and give it to her. So often we think nice things about others but never say them. And each time this happens we've missed a golden opportunity to increase our own, and other people's happiness.

I gave 20 UplifTin cards to a few friends for them to use with others, and the response was so great. I saw cards pop up in lunchboxes, teacher's desks, gift baskets, and slid into letterboxes. They created smiles, joy, and yes - they made the giver feel great as well as the receiver. You don't have to do anything huge. Just telling someone they look great or that they are an awesome friend is enough to boost spirits on both sides.

I say again: **Giving doesn't have to be a physical gift.** Giving is simply a way in which you can increase others' happiness, and your own as well. Giving isn't passive. It is an action. Something you have to actively do, for another. You are 'giving' joy. Here's another example:

My sister-in-law (the same one who loves giving gifts) is a teacher, and she started what she coined 'The Box of Awesomeness' at her workplace. Teachers nominate each other for big and little things such as handing in paperwork on time, a beautiful display, or demonstrating extra effort. At the beginning of every staff meeting they read the nominations out, the teachers get to pick from a prize box, and every meeting starts with happiness. How awesome is that! This is what I mean by giving.

It doesn't even matter how big or small your 'gift' is. Studies have shown that it is the act of giving, rather than the scale, or the amount of the gift, that makes the biggest difference. Have you heard that it is better to go on several small breaks throughout the year, rather than one big holiday? The small breaks make you just as relaxed, and because they are spread out throughout the year, that relaxation sticks around a lot longer.

In the same way, it would bring you more joy to give in smaller amounts over a year than to make one large donation, whether this is of your time or income. Volunteering once a month at a homeless shelter will buoy you more than a week solid once a year. As would donating just $5 to several worthy causes over a year rather than supporting one in a bigger way. Smaller gifts not only make you feel good about yourself more frequently, they give you an opportunity to show your support for multiple people or charities, sharing the love.

I recently took part in 'Shave for a Cure,' which is a fundraising event for the Leukemia Foundation. I shaved all my hair off (to no. 1 - eek!) and raised over $2000. It's still growing back, and while I don't love the look, I am so proud of myself. Giving my hair (I donated it for wigs) gave me confidence in myself and my abilities, a sense of self-worth, and made me feel great that I could support such a worthwhile cause.

And every time someone donated in the lead-up to the event, no matter how big or small, their gift lifted me up. I felt so loved, and it gave me the courage I needed to see it through. Since then I have had people message me or see me in person to say thank you. Many had struggled with cancer themselves in the past, and shaving my head not only raised awareness and money for research but helped them feel they weren't alone and that somebody cared.

I was almost bought to tears when my daughter's class all clapped for me when I came to help with their literacy groups (okay, I'm lying, I had tears). It got them talking and helped them understand what cancer sufferers go through. These are all things I never would have anticipated happening. The ripples of my actions are still continuing with several people inspired to participate in 'Shave for a Cure' next year, just as someone else inspired me. This one act of giving changed not just my look, but my whole life.

My friend does something similar in the US by donating her hair to "Locks of Love," an organization that makes wigs for young, disadvantaged cancer patients. Not only does it make her feel better about paying for the pampering of a salon day, it gives her warm fuzzies thinking of the good that gift is doing.

A word of caution. Giving can also be draining if you give more of yourself, your money, or your energy, than you can afford. A good example of this is a tithe. A tithe is similar to a tax which you give out of your wage to your church. It is often 10% of your earnings. This is less of a giving opportunity in most instances, and more of something that people feel compelled to do.

When you feel you *have* to do something, the joy connected with that gift is lost, and happiness levels can actually decrease. Giving is not about making grand gestures, or doing something on a permanent basis, so make sure that you are giving of yourself sustainably. Genuine giving is not about recognition, or accolades either. **True giving has no motivating factor behind it and requires nothing back. Giving should simply be about bringing joy into someone else's life.**

Your greatness is not what you have,
it's what you give.

Here's a list of things to give you some ideas on the giving front. There are infinite opportunities out there. Some can be planned, and some will be spontaneous. Just keep an eye out for them. Your mood will thank you, believe me!

Time

- Make a meal for someone who is sick
- Mow a neighbour's lawn
- Walk a friend's dog
- Spend uninterrupted time with your kids
- Help a friend with a task
- Volunteer somewhere
- Offer your skills
- Share your knowledge
- Routinely check in on someone
- Have someone over for a meal or a simple cuppa

Money

- Donate to someone's cause
- Give to the needy
- Sponsor a child
- Participate in a buy one give one meal order
- Support a group or organisation
- Support local endeavours
- Give your change to a busker
- Pay for someone's groceries
- Salary sacrifice for charity
- Shop at a local business instead of a big store
- Be more charitable
- Buy handmade

Support

- Give blood

- Pick litter up off the street

- Put yourself on the organ donation register

- Raise money for a good cause

- Organise a charity event

- Help a friend move house

- Offer your spot in a queue

- See a need, fill a need

- Tell someone they're doing a good job

- Mind someone's children or pets for them so they get a break

- Be there for a friend when they need you

Love

- Pay a compliment

- Make someone smile or laugh

- Give someone a call/a text/an email

- Support someone in a time of need

- Give a handwritten card even if it just says, 'You're awesome!'

- Be kind

- Forgive someone

- Pick a bunch of flowers for your neighbour

- Be encouraging

- Give the benefit of the doubt in tough situations

- Give someone your attention

- Listen when you're needed

- Build relationships with people 🔗 1

- Give your seat up for someone

- Say hello and smile at strangers. You may be the only person who has engaged with them that day.

- Be thoughtful

- Really 'see' people. Are they happy, healthy? Stop and ask yourself if you know what's happened in their lives this week. ASK them how they are. Listen.

Begin your day with thinking of one way you can give of your time, love, or money 🔗 2. Anticipate it - it's exciting! Do it - it will make you feel great. Reflect on it. What impact did that giving have on you, and on the recipient? One small act can change the whole way you look at your day. It is that powerful!

Often the little acts of giving we do are just what many would call the 'right thing to do.' And yet we've lost this instinctual 'rightness' somewhere along the way. And we need to remind ourselves, and others, that giving can, and should, be an integral, and instinctual part of our lives.

Giving in a positive way can help to improve your health, happiness, and self-worth. Giving can also remind us to be grateful for what we have and stops us dwelling on our own problems. Volunteering your time may help to keep our brains functioning well, which is great, because giving can even influence how long we live![66] It is truly remarkable what such a simple act can do for you, and those around you.

* * *

---

[66] http://psycnet.apa.org/record/2011-17888-001

RECAP 📌

- Giving is powerful! One small act of giving can change your whole day's perspective, increase the happiness of those around you, and increase your own as a by-product.

- Giving of our time, love, and energy helps create connections between people, which in turn can increase happiness.

- People you give to are more likely to give to others because of it. Your gift is like ripples in a pond, spreading indefinitely.

- Giving isn't passive, it's an action. Something you actively do for another. You are 'giving' joy.

- Studies have shown it is the act of giving, rather than the scale, or the amount of the gift, that makes the biggest difference.

- Genuine giving is not about recognition or accolades. It has no motivating factor behind it and requires nothing back. Giving should simply be about bringing joy into another person's life.

ACTION STEPS ✏️

Do now:

- Using the list above as a starting point, write your own list of giving. What are some things you can do in your day-to-day life to uplift, support, and bring joy to others?

- Use your list and find one thing you can do right now, to bring someone else happiness.

Plan to:

- Include giving in your daily life. Giving shouldn't be something that happens only on special occasions, but every day in small ways.

- Reflect on your giving so you can see what a big difference it makes in yours, and other peoples, lives.

Work towards:

- Doing something you've never done before. Whether it's shaving your hair off, volunteering at a homeless shelter, or doing a door knock appeal. Challenge yourself to give it a go, and then tell everyone what you're doing so you can't back out, and so they can support you. You will be amazed at how great you feel (even if you're a bit scared).

LINKED TO ⊚

1. Social Butterfly

2. Get Out of Bed You Daisy Head

UNPLUG YOUR BRAIN
♪♫♪ DANCING CRAZY — REYNA ARMOUR ♪♫♪

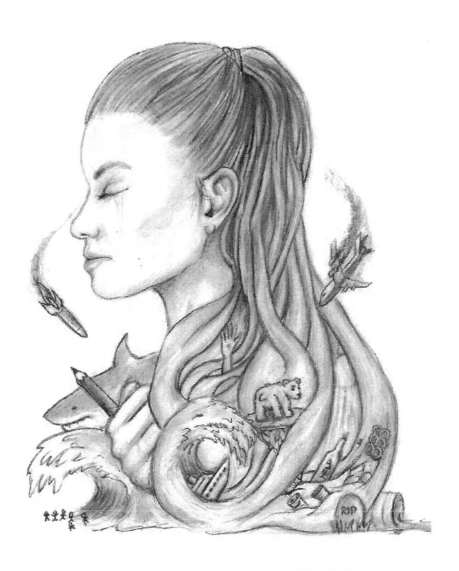

ARTWORK BY CRAIG DAWSON

We have never been more connected to the world around us than we are now. Social media, news reports, emails, calendar appointments. They all come to us in an instant via laptops, tablets, mobile phones, and smart watches. And even if you turn off all your notifications, the 6 o'clock news, radio broadcasts, and regular screen time will still keep you up to date. But is all this connection really a good thing?

It doesn't matter whether you love it or hate it, one thing is true. We can't control what we see when we open up a newspaper, turn on the radio, or scroll through a news feed. But we can control whether we listen to or read the media at all.

Let's face it. The news is mostly negative. People are killing each other, horrible things are happening, our world is dying, politicians are lying, humans are generally behaving far worse than animals, and it all seems to happen on a loop. Yes, I'm generalising.

Often, articles are written or reported from one person's or faction's view point. This means you usually get a distorted picture, instead of the whole one. Many blog posts and articles you see online are inaccurate and some are even downright lies, 'click-bait' aimed only at getting traffic.

Everything we see, read, and hear in our day has an impact on how we feel.

So, let me ask you this. Is keeping 'up to date' with news worth you feeling stressed and depressed? I used to feel guilty or stupid when I didn't know what was going on in the world around me, but then I realised my knowing about the bad things happening in the world was not changing them.

I can't fix the oil spill, the election, or stop the war. I wish I could, but I can't! If you really want to enable change, then find something you *can* help with, and make it happen! 🖉 1 Set up a community alert so you know about local things like clean up days. Join the SES and help people out after natural disasters. Research reputable sources and then vote knowledgably on election day. These are things you can actively do to bring about positive change, and very few of them are discovered by reading or listening to secular news.

When I stopped listening to the news, the conversations I had with people actually became much more meaningful, because we talked about the things that were happening in our own worlds rather than in others'.

It didn't matter that I wasn't up to date on who won the Oscars, which world leader was being tried for a crime, and how much money our government had wasted on another useless venture. I found I got to know not only other people, but myself, and what was important to me, better. I also found I had a more balanced understanding of the things that did interest or affect me, because instead of listening to and reading biased reports, I did my own research.

I do feel it's important to know about large changes that can affect you and those you love. And you may need to keep on top of certain aspects of the news for your job. This could include natural disasters, countries invading one another (this happens a surprising amount...), local elections and reforms. However, you don't have to read the news for an hour a day to receive this information. Here's some ways you can stay informed without becoming overwhelmed.

- Look at online news headlines from reputable sources, and then choose which ones may be important enough for you to read.

- Put a time limit on your news intake.

- Don't read the news when you first wake up, as it can set your mood for the day. And not in a good way. ⌬ 2

- Don't read it before you go to bed either, when it can disrupt sleep.

- Get a housemate, friend, or family member to keep you informed of big events.

- Listen to the hourly news bulletins on your local radio station. These are normally only a few minutes long and only have the main headlines. Plus, you'll get the weather report, which is always good.

- Use your work's Intranet to stay informed about topical news.

Some media outlets are catching on. One station my friend listens to features a segment in their morning show called "Tell Me Something Good." The stories they share might come from local or national news, or even be good news about someone that one of the DJs is acquainted with. It happens to broadcast just before she leaves for work, and not only is it a lovely change-up from the usual doom and gloom, it can help boost her mood for the day ahead. If you can find a segment like this, then by all means – listen!

On top of the mental effects of media, there has been countless research done into the ways technology affects us physically. Things like Wi-Fi signals, and the blue light from computer and plasma TV screens, are all under investigation for disrupting your brain patterns, and causing awesome things like insomnia, irritability, and depression. ⌬ 3

While many people say that Wi-Fi signals are not strong enough to cause any adverse effects, studies where plants are grown next to Wi-Fi and in a Wi-Fi free zone show vastly different results.

☢ Six girls at Hjallerup School in Denmark designed an experiment that would test the effect of cell phone radiation on a plant. The students placed six trays filled with Lepidium sativum, a type of garden cress, into a room without radiation, and six trays of the seeds into another room next to two routers that according to the girls' calculations, emitted about the same type of radiation as an ordinary cell phone.[68] By the end of the experiment the results were blatantly obvious — the cress seeds placed near the router had not grown. Many of them were completely dead. Meanwhile, the cress seeds planted in the other room, away from the routers, thrived.

Look at moving all electronic devices out of your bedroom, or at the very least switching off Wi-Fi while you sleep. Try to minimize your time spent on devices, and in front of the television, especially for that hour before bed. Instead, swap screen time for 'green time' (time outdoors).

We've become so reliant on technology and spend so much time plugged into varying forms of tech, that what little time we have left after work and other chores is being consumed, making it harder to connect on a personal level with others, and even ourselves.

One of the saddest things I've ever seen was when I used to work at IKEA. We had a 700-seat restaurant, and it was always

---

[68] http://www.waldorftoday.com/2013/07/student-science-experiment-finds-plants-wont-grow-near-wi-fi-router/

busy. One night I noticed a grandmother, mother, and two children having dinner together around one of our family tables. It would have been a nice scene, except every single one of them was on a device. The grandmother was on an iPad. The mum was on her phone, and the two children were playing computer games. Dinner is supposed to be a social time, where you talk to each other, and find out how everyone's day has been. ✍ 4 This family weren't even making eye contact. I mean, what was the frickin' point of going out to eat?

TV is another shining example.

> ☢ "Emotional content of films and television programs can affect your psychological health. It can do this by directly affecting your mood, and your mood can then affect many aspects of your thinking and behavior. If the TV program generates negative mood experiences (e.g., anxiety, sadness, anger, disgust), then these experiences will affect how you interpret events in your own life, what types of memories you recall, and how much you will worry about events in your own life."[69]

I know it's a bit much to ask you not to watch TV at all, but think about *diminishing* your television consumption. **The average American watches a shocking 5 hours of television a day.**

5 hours! What the heck! And two-thirds watch television while they're having dinner[70]. There's an easy way to cut back and reconnect with your family right there.

---

[69] https://www.psychologytoday.com/blog/why-we-worry/201206/the-psychological-effects-tv-news
[70] https://www.statisticbrain.com/television-watching-statistics/

☢ "TV doesn't really seem to satisfy people over the long haul the way that social involvement or reading a newspaper does. We looked at eight to ten activities that happy people engage in, and for each one, the people who did the activities more — visiting others, going to church, all those things — were more happy. TV was the one activity that showed a negative relationship. Unhappy people did it more, and happy people did it less. The data suggest to us that the TV habit may offer short-run pleasure at the expense of long-term malaise." [71]

And while you're at it, your gaming on computers, phones, or tablets has the same effect as TV. While it won't harm you in small amounts, the sheer volume most people use their devices is debilitating both mentally and physically. And I'm not just talking about eye strain either. Studies indicate that spending significant amounts of time in front of a screen (that's any screen) can have a massive impact on your cardiovascular health and your mortality. Yup - you die earlier. And this is still true even if you exercise! ▶

Kick the kids outside or use that free time to play a board game, create something arty or crafty, write a letter, listen to a podcast, practice meditation ✎ 5, talk to your partner (heaven forbid!), visit a friend for an evening cuppa, or go really wild and do something for yourself like read a book, take a bubble bath, or journal.

Changing your evenings from time in front of the TV to time spent creating, connecting ✎ 6, or relaxing ✎ 7 will make a huge difference in your happiness. You will feel less rushed, more energetic, and more connected with those around you.

---

[71] https://www.psychologytoday.com/us/blog/inner-source/201110/your-unhappy-brain-television -Robinson J. 2008 Social Indicators Research

You don't have to make big changes. You can start by cutting out one show a week and go from there.

"The remarkable thing about television is that it permits several million people to laugh at the same joke and still feel lonely."
-T.S. ELIOT-

Technology is awesome, don't get me wrong. I 'ask Google' so many things I swear I should own shares in the company. And like all things, it can be a good thing when used correctly. It is a great way to reach out to people if you are too scared or anxious to do so in person. It makes it easy for people to stay in touch, and to set up face-to-face fun, and there are some really awesome apps and games available for those struggling with sadness, anxiety, and mental health issues.

Used the right way, technology can be not only helpful, but healing. Unfortunately, the majority of technology use is anything but healing. Use the suggestions in this chapter to turn your use of television, tablets and computers into tools that increase your happiness, rather than contributing to your low mood.

* * *

RECAP

- We are more connected than ever before, and everything we see, read, or hear has an impact on how we feel.

- We can't control what we see or hear on mainstream media, but we can control if we listen to or read it at all.

- You don't have to read the news for an hour a day to receive the information you need. Use simple hacks to stay informed without becoming overwhelmed.

- Changing your evenings from time spent in front of the TV to time spent creating, connecting, or relaxing will make a huge difference to your happiness.

ACTION STEPS ✎

Do now:

- Write a list of all the things you enjoy doing and see which ones you could do in the time you normally spend reading news, watching television, and using technology.

Plan to:

- Cut back your time gaming or in front of the television by 15 minutes a week.

- Get relevant news from reliable sources and use at least one hack to limit how much time you spend on media.

Work towards:

- Using technology for good things such as learning and connecting with others.

- Watching TV or using screens for only a small portion of your day

- Switching off whenever you can

LINKED TO

1. Give a Little

2. Get Out of Bed You Daisy Head

3. Successful Slumber

4. Eat the Food!

5. Meditation is for Weirdos

6. Social Butterfly

7. Relaxation is a Real Thing

LIKE, COMMENT, SHARE
♪♫♪ DANZA KUDURO – DON OMAR FT LUCENZO ♪♫♪

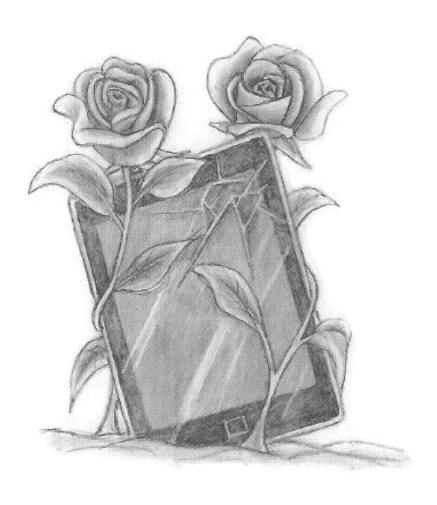

ARTWORK BY CRAIG DAWSON

No one's perfect. But with the rise of social media, we are often left feeling so much 'less' than others, because we are constantly comparing ourselves to them. The crazy thing about this is that we don't know their whole story. We don't see behind the scenes, but only a snapshot. What they want us to see.

And of course, those 'snapshots' they choose to share with us are the 'perfect' ones. Who wants to show the world their bad moments? The tears, the tantrums, the ugly days, the days that just fell apart, the debt drowning them because of that amazing holiday they took. Nobody shows the world that crap! So, the only things we are comparing ourselves to are the magical (and often staged) moments they allow us to see.

> *"Don't compare your insides with other people's outsides."*

I challenge you to #showustherealpicture on Facebook, Instagram and Twitter. I want to see the photo of your child having a meltdown. I want to see the dress you can't zip up. I want to see your car broken down on the side of the road. I want to see you working a public holiday so you can afford to buy a house. I want to see the run you took that allows you to eat burgers and still look great. (It's not magic, people) This is the action behind the scenes. What makes up the real-life version of yourself. Because this is the true picture.

If we compared ourselves to this truer picture of others, we would see that everyone has good days and bad days. Not everyone is loaded, living it up large, or loving their job. Not everyone looks amazing the moment they roll out of bed. Some days we sit in our PJ's and watch movies because we don't want to do anything else. And that's ok! This is the real picture!

Dwelling on what we don't have in our lives, rather than what we do have, makes it so much harder to be happy. Learning to accept that we are all different people, living different lives at different speeds, makes it so much easier to simply live, love, and enjoy our own lives 🖉 1. Whereas constantly comparing ourselves to others on social media, makes it almost impossible.

And don't even get me started on the *time* we waste on social media.

> ✸ The average person will spend nearly two hours on social media every day, which translates to a total of 5 years and 4 months spent over a lifetime. Currently, total time spent on social media beats time spent eating and drinking, socializing, and grooming, and is only surpassed by TV. And it's only expected to increase as platforms develop.[72]

I used to waste a *lot* of time on social media, and it's still something I'm constantly working on improving. You go on Facebook to check on that 'work-related post,' and half an hour later you get off knowing about 21 ways to clean up stains, what people you don't really know did over the weekend, and what colour your personality is. And, you've missed the only window you had to go for a run.

Social media can be awesome. It's fantastic for keeping in touch with people, both locally and overseas. It allows you to share moments in your life that make you happy, and proud, and it

---

[72] http://www.socialmediatoday.com/marketing/how-much-time-do-people-spend-social-media-infographic

can be a great marketing tool for businesses. However, very few people are self-controlled enough to make it work for them, instead of being worked by it. And social media, instead of bringing people closer, can actually distance you from friends.

Say you've know a girl called Emma for several years. She's not a close friend, but you used to catch up every few months for a coffee and a chat. Now you only bump into her at mutual friends' parties. Why? Because by going on Facebook and liking her posts, commenting when something awesome or sad happens, and seeing her selfies, you feel like you've already 'caught up.' You know what Emma's been up to. You've seen her holiday pics (lucky duck), and you know she's engaged. What else do you have to talk about? Facebook, instead of bringing you closer, has effectively shattered any chance of deepening your friendship, because you no longer feel you have to see her in person.

A good friend of mine has the right idea. She has a Facebook account, and she posts things on it occasionally, but if she goes to her feed, nothing comes up. While she has remained friends with all her contacts, she has 'unfollowed' them, which means when she logs in she is not distracted by an endless stream of comments and media. She has to physically click on a person to see what they've been up to.

Not only does this mean she doesn't get sucked into scrolling ever onwards, she also gets to decide what information, from whom, she is reading. She is my hero. 2

While you don't have to go to that extreme, here are a few tips on getting control of your social media addiction.

- Set specific times for looking at social media and set an alarm. Don't look at it outside this time.

- If you want to upload something, write a note and do it in your set time.

- Set a timer for 10 minutes each time you open a social media page. Get off as soon as it sounds.

- If you find you've been scrolling for a while get up, do 5-star jumps, and then see if what you were reading was important enough to sit back down for.

- Ask yourself if what you're reading/watching/commenting on is teaching you anything about yourself, your friends, or your world. Honestly.

- Check your goals ✪ 3 list for the day and see if you've completed them... Stop procrastinating!

- Take social media apps off your phone and tablet. Having to work that little bit harder to access them means you're not clicking on them out of boredom.

- Turn off all notifications!!

Unfortunately, social media addiction is not helped by how connected we all are. Phones, the ever present, always on, 'asset' owned by almost everyone, are not only linked to our social media accounts, but set up to alert us of any and all interactions. But what effect are they really having on our lives?

Always having something to do in our downtime means the brain is struggling to process new information and create memories out of it. And the sheer fact that we are constantly 'switched on' is making us all stressed.

> 😵 We don't attempt to store information in our own memory to the same degree that we used to, because we know that the Internet knows everything... One could speculate that this extends to personal memories, as constantly looking at the world through the lens of our smartphone camera may result in us trusting our smartphones to store our memories for us. This way, we pay less attention to life itself and become worse at remembering events from our own lives. [73]

If you accidentally leave your phone at home, and you have even a few minutes where you are sitting quietly without distraction, what do you do?

I fidget. I'm so used to using my phone in quiet moments, I've forgotten how to be still. And I'm not the only one! I've started to deliberately leave my phone at home, so I can re-learn how to be alone, without the need for constant entertainment and connection. And you know what? When used in concert with breathing ◎ 4 and mindfulness ◎ 5, it is so damn relaxing!

Not only that, but when you're not staring at a phone, you are more likely to engage in conversations with real, live people. What the heck! Talking - to real people?

Having our heads down staring at screens effectively signals to people that we are busy and don't want to be disturbed. Often though, we are just bored and filling time. We no longer strike up conversations and build friendships with 'random' people, because we are effectively removing ourselves from any situations where we could, by absorbing ourselves with social media. ◎ 6

---

[73] Dr. Maria Wimber, University of Birmingham

Life is all about our experiences, and many of those are built around the people we meet. Often randomly! I have had many conversations with people that ended up turning into friendships which have lasted years. And even if your chat is simply that, most times you will leave with a smile, a wave, and an increase in happiness. Even if it's just a chuckle about how crazy that person just was!

Learn a bit of phone etiquette. This means putting your phone away while talking to a person. Especially when it's your children. Don't go up to a salesperson while you're still talking on your phone. And definitely don't watch Facebook videos while you're having a conversation! We've all been guilty of some of these things, but they are so flippin' rude! You are effectively telling the person you're talking to that what you're doing on the phone is more important than they are.

Try switching off all the notifications for your phone and don't forget your smart watch if you have one. You will have less distractions, and you'll get to spend a lot more time on important things. If you're struggling to break the habit of looking at your phone, install a learning, ⌀7 mindfulness, or mood app and use it to better your life, instead of inundating yourself with the often-destructive media at your fingertips. Learn to disconnect from social media and reconnect with life.

* * *

RECAP ⚷

- Social media doesn't give us the whole picture, but only a snapshot of people's lives, and usually only the positive aspects.

- Comparing yourself to others makes it almost impossible to live, love, and enjoy your own life.

- Social media can be fantastic; however, few people are self-controlled enough to make it work for them, rather than being worked by it.

- Learning phone etiquette and switching off notifications, can open you up to new experiences and friendships, and put you more in touch with yourself.

- #showustherealpicture on Facebook, Instagram, and Twitter and help others see that their chaos is actually the norm!

ACTION STEPS ✎

Do now:

- Write a list of all the things you enjoy doing and see which ones you could do in the time you normally spend on social media. You will be amazed at how much you can free up your day.

- Do something wild like deleting social media apps off your phone, or unfollowing people on Facebook. What!

Plan to:

- Limit your social media time and avoid it altogether early in the morning ⊘8 and before bed at night. ⊘9

- Leave your phone at home next time you go for a walk.

- Post some *real* photos with the #showustherealpicture hashtag.

- Have phone-free zones. At the dinner table, picking your child up from school, catching up with friends, to name but a few.

Work towards:

- Not looking at your phone in a public setting

- Using mindfulness and breathing exercises in place of social media when you're bored

- Switching off whenever you can

LINKED TO

1. Great Attitude

2. Unplug Your Brain

3. Aim for the Stars

4. Breathe and Pose

5. Mind Your Mind

6. Social Butterfly

7. Learning to Grow

8. Get Out of Bed You Daisy Head

9. Successful Slumber

LEARNING TO GROW
♪♫♪ SEND ME ON MY WAY — RUSTED ROOT ♪♫♪

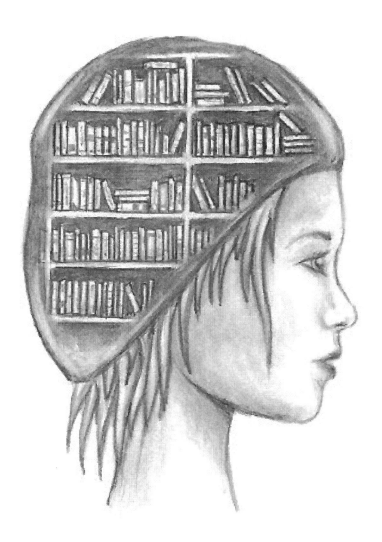

ARTWORK BY CRAIG DAWSON

Learning new skills and gaining knowledge affects our wellbeing in lots of positive ways. It exposes us to new ideas and helps us stay curious and engaged. It offers us opportunities to meet new people, and experience things we may not have otherwise. It also gives us a sense of accomplishment and helps boost our self-confidence and resilience.

There are a limitless number of ways to learn and grow in our lives. We can attend a course and learn a new skill through formal education. We can learn from friends, family members, or community members. We can join a club, a sporting group, or attend an event. Whatever you enjoy, there will be others out there who enjoy the same things. Get on the Internet and on social media and seek them out. If you join and it doesn't seem to be quite the right fit, find another one, or start your own! How do you think clubs begin in the first place?

When you join a group, ensure you are giving it a good shot, even if you're shy. Are you initiating conversations? Don't automatically think that because people don't talk to you, they don't like you. Other people can be shy too, remember. If you're freaking out, try using one of the approaches we discuss in 'Social Butterfly' 1- especially the power of 'one.' Give it a good crack. It takes a while for new things to go from being scary and awkward to enjoyable.

If you really don't think you're up to joining a club, you don't have to. The Internet has brought the world to your doorstep in such a way that you don't even have to leave the house to learn new skills if you don't want to. You can take an online course, watch a tutorial on YouTube, or download and read books on a topic you're interested in.

There is simply no reason not to be continuously learning. Oh, you'll hear them all at some point, but most people's 'reasons' are really their excuses. Many types of learning are free, so cost is not truly a barrier (think the library and the Internet). There are also many community groups that are free of charge. I am part of a local running group that I don't pay a cent for, and which along with providing me with great social interaction, has taught me a lot about my body and my endurance.

Time isn't an excuse either. It's simply something we need to make better use of. I get it, you're busy. We all are. But you don't have to do hours of learning a day to get the positive effects of it. You can try something new or actively seek out knowledge for only half an hour a day and still create massive growth in your life.

TV, social media, and an overabundance of 'stuff' in our lives all contribute to a lack of time, but things like books and flashcards are very easy to take with you for whenever you have a spare moment. After-school activities, work functions, and lunch hours can all become learning opportunities.

You can even listen to podcasts or tuitions while you work or commute. And did you know that when you listen to foreign language recordings while you sleep it actually helps you learn?[74] While you sleep! How easy is that for time-poor people? It's all about making the best use of your time. See 'Sort Your Crazy' ⊘ 2 to help you put the important things first.

I feel a lot of the time we don't learn new things because it would mean putting ourselves out there to be judged by others, and to potentially fail. We are so conditioned by society that life is all about winning that we never try, in case we don't succeed. This is incredibly sad, because if we never try anything new,

---

[74] https://academic.oup.com/cercor/article/25/11/4169/2366428

and never challenge ourselves, we will never grow and evolve as a person.

> *"When my brother and I were growing up, my father would encourage us to fail. We'd sit around the dinner table and he'd ask, "What did you guys fail at this week?" If we had nothing to tell him, he'd be disappointed. My father wanted us to try everything, and feel free to push the envelope."*
>
> -SARA BLAKELY-

If you're worried about failing, then learn how to rejection proof yourself▶. Sara Blakely, the founder of Spanx (and also a billionaire), grew up doing this.

And it is precisely this type of outlook that can change your life. It doesn't matter if you try something and you hate it! It doesn't matter if you fail miserably! And it doesn't even matter if you're so embarrassed you want to sink into the ground. Give things a shot, because the positives will always outweigh the negatives. Even if you can't see them at the time.

I was 16 when I left home to go to college quite a long way away. It was the first time I had really been out in the world by myself, and I learned an incredible amount about myself in a short space of time. I learned coping skills, how to be responsible for myself, and I found out I was terrible with money! I generally grew up a lot, and I changed.

And I think I changed for the better. But it only happened because I got out of my comfort zone and tried something new. Simply put, when you don't put yourself out there, you don't learn or grow as a person.

Change is a part of human nature, and even change that at the time might not be brilliant, still moulds you into you. **People who never put themselves in new situations never grow as a person. And they never learn the self-satisfaction, the pride, and the gratification that comes with getting out there and giving something a shot.** Yes, it can be daunting, yes, it can be hard, and yes, you may fail. But it can also be incredibly rewarding and bring you an insane amount of happiness.

How? One of the reasons humans are at the top of the food chain is through evolution. No matter what you believe we started as, a blob of goo or formed by the hand of God, it is irrefutable that we as a species evolve over the ages. If we didn't, our growth would have stagnated, and we would have remained in the Stone Age forever.

Humans (and animals) evolve through change. In fact, to evolve simply means to change. And one of the biggest contributing factors to change is learning.

> *"If we don't change, we don't grow. If we don't grow, we aren't really living."*
> -GAIL SHEEHY-

Warren Buffet (one of the most successful investors of all time and a self-made billionaire) estimates he spends 80% of his day reading and learning. He talks about how learning every day builds knowledge, and that knowledge then accumulates like compound interest. His business partner Charlie Munger says, "Go to bed smarter than when you woke up."

You don't have to do anything catastrophic. Don't know how to spell a word? Look it up. Want to know why the sky is blue? Me too! Look it up.

The Internet has made knowledge so accessible that there is no excuse for you not to learn at least one new thing every day. And these little learnings are awesome! But the more you put yourself out there, the bigger the rewards.

Challenge yourself, and you will be surprised at what you can accomplish. Don't think you're smart enough to learn new things? Think again! Every single person has the capacity to learn. Your brain is flexible, and not only is it possible to continue learning throughout your life, but imperative for good brain function.

> ☻ Neurologist and educator Judy Willis encourages lifelong learning and says: "Especially for students who believe they are 'not smart,' the realization that they can literally change their brains through study and review is empowering."[75]

Trying new things not only opens us up to new experiences but ensures that we are always growing as a person, and this in turn makes you a happier, more well-rounded person who can look back on their life and say, "I tried so many interesting things." Even the crazy, catastrophic ones will be good for a giggle!

---

[75] https://www.edutopia.org/neuroscience-brain-based-learning-neuroplasticity

Harry Potter wouldn't exist if JK Rowling hadn't put herself out there over and over again. I mean, come on, people! What would a world without Hogwarts be like?

You don't have to change the world, but if you create change in your life you will never look back. It is hard to be happy when you live your life on repeat, so try something new, and grow as a person. You won't regret it.

* * *

RECAP ✂

- Learning new skills, and gaining knowledge exposes us to new ideas, and helps us stay curious and engaged. It also gives us a sense of accomplishment and helps boost our self-confidence and resilience.

- Many types of learning are free, so cost is not truly a barrier. Think of your local library or community centre, the Internet or YouTube.

- You can try something new or actively seek out knowledge for only half an hour a day and still create massive growth in your life.

- When you don't learn, you don't grow as a person. Challenge yourself, and you'll be surprised at what you can accomplish.

- Your brain is flexible, and even if you believe you're not 'smart,' you still have the capacity and ability to learn.

ACTION STEPS ✎

Do now:

Reflect on the past few months and answer these questions:

- What have you learnt or tried out for the first time recently?

- How did it make you feel?

- Do you think it has altered your perspective of yourself or your world?

- Did you enjoy it?

- Would you do it again?

- Why don't you try new things? Lack of time, money, confidence?

- What can you do to combat this?

- What have you always wanted to do or try?

Now write a list of new things you could try over the next few months. It could be something simple, or a more complex idea, like:

- Taking a different route to work

- Reading a different newspaper

- Visiting a local spot you've never quite got to

- Learning first aid

- Learning a language

- Trying out for a sports team,

- Signing up for a charity event

- Feeling part of something bigger by engaging physically or through social media

- Doing something outside of your comfort zone

- Visiting an inspiring location

- Gazing at the stars one evening

- Looking up the meaning of words you don't know

- Joining a club

- Trying a new recipe

- Literally anything else you can think of!

Plan to:

- Each week try to include one new learning opportunity into your life. ◎3 It may be something little, or something big. It's up to you. Try to make it something you're genuinely interested in though, so you look forward to it.

- Say yes to things you would normally say no to. Sometimes new experiences and learning opportunities come from the most unlikely sources!

- Reflect on what you've done each week, and see how it's changed your attitude, your outlook on life, and your joy and appreciation of the world around you. Would you have done anything differently?

Work towards:

- Including at least half an hour of learning into your day. This might be through formal learning, or simply through reading, online browsing, or hands-on skills.

- Actively putting yourself into situations you find scary. Fear is a great catalyst for change and growth. If it's not scary then you know you're not stretching yourself as much as you could be. Put yourself out there! You'll be amazed at what you can achieve.

LINKED TO

1. Social Butterfly

2. Sort Your Crazy

3. Aim for the Stars

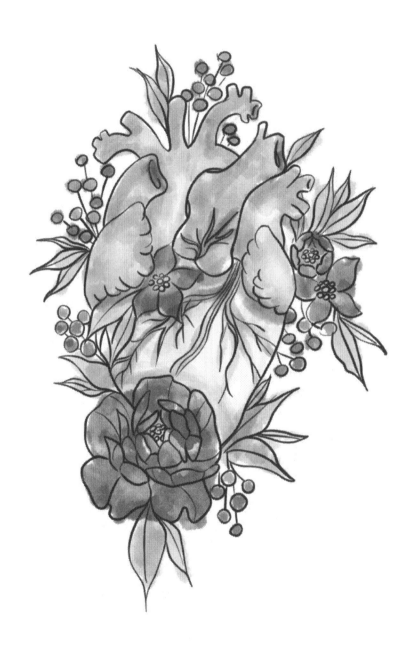

ARTWORK BY RACHEL "WOLVES"

SELF

CHANGING YOUR INNER SELF CAN OFTEN BE HARDER THAN ALTERING YOUR PHYSICAL BODY. YOU CAN'T 'SEE' THE CHANGES, INSTEAD THEY ARE CHARACTERIZED BY HOW YOU SEE, REACT AND PROCESS ALL THE LITTLE THINGS THAT MAKE UP LIFE.

AND YET INSPECTING YOUR VALUES AND BELIEF SYSTEMS, LEARNING GRATITUDE AND MINDFULNESS, AND KNOWING HOW TO SMILE WHEN YOU LEAST FEEL LIKE IT, ARE SOME OF THE MOST IMPORTANT CHANGES YOU CAN MAKE.

SPIRITUAL VALUE
♪♫♪ CAN'T STOP THE FEELING – JUSTIN TIMBERLAKE ♪♫♪

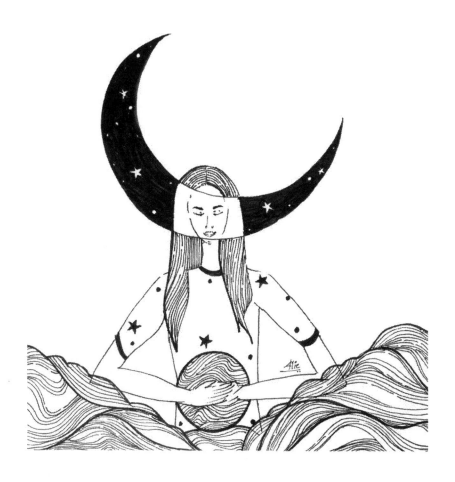

ARTWORK BY 4LIE_ARTWORKS

The meaning of spirituality is in the word itself. It is about your spirit, your soul, the very essence of your being, rather than material or physical things.

Everything from the values and beliefs you grew up with, your environment, your religious affiliations, and your core beliefs, can form part of your spirituality. It means different things to different people, but spirituality, no matter what form it takes, always provides people with meaning and joy in their lives and helps balance them.

Spirituality, for you, may not have anything to do with a God, or a religious belief. Perhaps spirituality for you is walking in nature, or volunteering for a cause. It could be uplifting others in a time of need, or simply being the best person you can possibly be. I feel far more in tune with myself, or 'spiritual' if you like, by listening to waves break on the beach than I do sitting in a church.

Check out the list below and see which actions you relate to the most. Each one can form a part of your life's spirituality. They all, on one level or another, help you to become more attuned with yourself, and the very core of your being. They can help reset the inner you and nourish your spirit and soul. This, more than any belief others may expect you to hold, is spirituality.

- Yoga
- Meditation ✪1
- Prayer
- Dance ✪2
- Painting
- Practicing gratitude ✪3
- Philosophy
- Giving to others of your time, support, or friendship ✪4

- Attending religious meetings
- Running
- Walking in nature
- Learning
- Contemplating the world around you.
- Doing nothing but sitting, looking, listening, smelling, and feeling.

All these things can help different people at different stages of their life, but like anything else, need to be practiced regularly. If surfing is your thing, then get out and surf before work! (Like you need another excuse.) If it is being part of your community through the giving of your time, then stop waiting for an opportunity to present itself and search one out!

If spirituality for you means attending a religious service each week, then really be present. Not because you need to be seen to be, but because that is what nourishes you as a person.

Religion and spirituality offer people support in the form of a sense of community, and a buffer in tough times. They can give you a sense of purpose, a goal to aim for, and help you feel in control of your life. If happiness is about being content with ourselves and our lives, then spirituality is a tool we can use to help get us there.

And yet spirituality is a personal journey. While you can take it alongside others, no one can decide what makes you feel whole. Only you know what your spirit needs. *All Blacks Don't Cry* author John Kirwin says it incredibly well.

"Philosophy, Shintoism, Zen, and Confucius are all spiritual. Core issues of life such as happiness, courage, ambition, regret and how to live a good life. All religions and philosophies have something to teach us. I look for lessons in life that I can apply to myself to make my life richer and more wholesome. Every situation that arises can be a learning situation."

-JOHN KIRWIN-▶

Nourishing your soul is about finding balance between the busyness of life, and the things that recharge us and bring us happiness. Be honest with yourself. Don't just think that because you were bought up with specific cultural expectations, or spiritual beliefs, that those are the things your soul craves now. Humans have an incredible ability to change and grow. And our beliefs on spirituality can change right along with us.

Many people let their spirituality stagnate. They decide early on they are going to follow a particular set of beliefs, and instead of using those beliefs to grow, they simply use them as a label. Just another way of fitting into the world's expectations of us.

We all know it is far more important to be ourselves than to follow the crowd, and yet spirituality, something that is so important in our lives, and in our ability to be truly happy, is something we let others decide for us, often from birth!

Spirituality has the ability to transform your life by offering a connection to something greater than yourself. It doesn't matter whether that something is nature, God, Buddha, or simply a community of like-minded people.

> ☻ Spirituality is linked to many important aspects of human functioning - spiritual people have positive relationships, high self-esteem, are optimistic, and have meaning and purpose in life. Spiritual individuals strive toward a better life and consider personal growth and fulfillment as a central goal. Spirituality can be considered to be a path toward self-actualization, because it requires people to focus on their internal values and work on becoming a better individual.[76]

No matter what you discover, or what form your spirituality takes, make sure it is a true representation of *your* beliefs, and not of others. Ask yourself some tough questions, take a really good look at yourself, and embrace the things that *you* need to be whole, peaceful, and happy. Without worrying about what other people think. That's their journey. This is yours!

*　　*　　*

RECAP ✄

- Spirituality is about your spirit, your soul, the very essence of your being, rather than material or physical things.

- Everything from the values and beliefs you grew up with, to your religious and core beliefs, can form part of your spirituality.

---

[76] https://www.psychologytoday.com/us/blog/cant-buy-happiness/201302/why-be-spiritual-five-benefits-spirituality

- No matter what form spirituality takes, it is always a personal journey. It helps balance people and provides them with meaning and joy in their lives.

- Actions you take help reset the inner you, nourish your spirit and soul, and become more attuned with yourself. These actions could be as varied as attending religious meetings to going for a surf.

- Many people let their spirituality stagnate or allow others to dictate their beliefs. No matter what form your spirituality takes, make sure it is a true representation of yourself.

ACTION STEPS ✎

Do now:

Start by asking yourself some questions on your philosophy for life and be honest with your answers. I've listed some good starters below. Use your answers, and the list of actions above, to help you decide what nourishes your soul. It may be one thing, it may be many. What makes you feel at peace, on an even keel, and true to yourself? Write it all down.

- What does spirituality mean to you?

- How do you want to live your life? Not how do you want to be *seen* to be living, but how do YOU want to live?

- What do you need to do every day to make that a reality?

- If you look back on your life, what things really helped nourish and sustain you as a person? Not your body, but your inner self.

- Do you want to leave the world a better place on your death? In what way? How can you make this happen?

- What brings you peace, joy, and contentment? How can you get more of it in your life?

Plan to:

- Work at least one spirituality action into your life every week.

- If you aren't sure what makes you feel whole, then start exploring spirituality and its meaning for you. Attend a church service, a yoga retreat, a philosophy or ethics discussion. Take a dance or art class, or simply be still in nature. Use the questions above to really hone in on what supports and nourishes the inner you.

Work towards:

- Introducing a spiritual action into your life daily.

- Growing your spirituality and leaving your comfort zone, so that you don't stagnate but instead flourish, grow, and truly know yourself.

LINKED TO

1. Meditation is for Weirdos

2. Create a Song and Dance

3. Great Attitude

4. Give a Little

SMILE – YOUR FACE WON'T CRACK
♪♫♪ SMILE – UNCLE KRAKER ♪♫♪

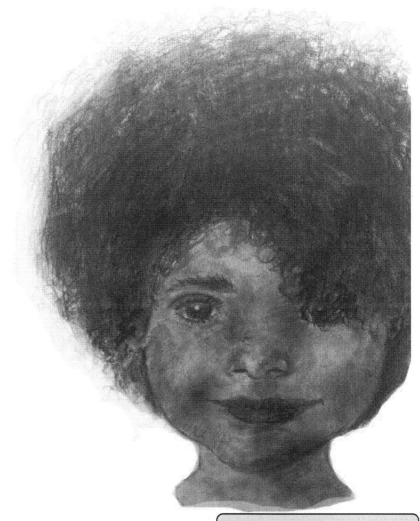

ARTWORK BY SAMANTHA OLIVIA SWAT

> *"I will never understand the good*
> *that a simple smile can accomplish."*
> -MOTHER TERESA-

Did you know we are born smiling? It is one of our most basic functions as human beings. We smile while still developing in the womb, we smile while sleeping once we're born, and all cultures use the smile to show joy and satisfaction. Crazy, right? Surely one forgotten or hidden tribe would use the smile to signify something else entirely. And yet they don't[77]. Because smiling changes your biochemistry and instantly puts you in a more positive state. Why would you use it to convey anything other than the joy you feel!

And yet somewhere over the course of our lives we stop. We forget to smile. We learn to suppress them, and instead school our faces to reflect the stressed, angry, sad, and serious faces of those around us. This is how we feel we are supposed to look. But why? People who smile are seen as more beautiful, competent, and likeable, so why do we put on this mask and call it adulthood?

Sometimes I think it's because we worry about others' perceptions of us. What they think, based on our outward appearance. We want people to know we are sad, worried, stressed, or angry without having to talk about it, so we change our faces to reflect what we want them to see. Unfortunately, all this does is make sure the feelings that may otherwise have been dealt with quickly stick around. By not encouraging happiness, we're embracing sadness.

---

[77] https://1ammce38pkj41n8xkp1iocwe-wpengine.netdna-ssl.com/wp-content/uploads/2013/07/Universal-Facial-Expressions-Of-Emotion.pdf

😊 Kids have got the right idea. They smile up to 400 times a day, in comparison to some adults who smile less than five times a day![78]

Science has proven that smiling makes you healthier by increasing your happiness hormones and decreasing your stress-enhancing hormones and can even help you live longer! It's not just about you though. When you give someone a smile it is almost impossible for them not to return it. People's whole attitudes and perspectives can alter, and they instantly feel happier.

You see, it is incredibly hard to frown when you are looking at someone who is smiling (although many people still like to practice it!). You must have seen the video clips of people on trains starting a contagious laugh. It spreads like wildfire and soon people are laughing for no apparent reason other than the fact that it brings them joy, and they can't seem to help it. Smiling is the same. It is contagious!

When we're feeling down, and don't feel like smiling, we assume we can't. But we've got it backwards. **It's not good feelings that make us smile, it's smiles that make us feel good!** What do I mean? It's like this. If you are hanging out with friends, having a good time, it's easy to smile and to laugh. But it's not just our friends making us feel good (although socialization ⊘ 1 is an important factor) it's smiling. It's a bit like the 'which came first, the chicken or the egg' scenario.

---

[78] https://www.forbes.com/sites/ericsavitz/2011/03/22/the-untapped-power-of-smiling/#4d310df77a67

The happiness of being with friends prompts us to smile, but it's the physical act of smiling itself that gives us that burst of good feelings. This means smiling is especially important if you are feeling down. When I first started to claw my way out of depression, I gave myself the challenge to smile every time I thought about it. It was incredibly hard at first and I even resorted to pushing the corners of my mouth up into an awful rictus of a smile. But you know what? Even that made me feel better! And the more often I smiled, the easier it became.

I learnt how to smile even when I was really angry or frustrated, and it helped immensely in calming me down, helping me see the funny side of situations, and even just allowing me to pause, and see the situation from a different perspective. It changed my mood far more than I ever thought it would. And faking a smile or a laugh is just as effective at lifting your mood as the real thing![79] Seriously.

Smiling is the single easiest, cheapest, solution to low mood and is available to everyone, everywhere, anytime. And remember, this is something we were born knowing how to do! We don't have to learn it, we just have to remember it!

Try it now. I challenge you to smile, a big goofy smile with your teeth showing, and not feel even a tiny bit better. Sometimes my daughter asks me, "Why are you smiling, Mum? Did you read something funny?" And I just say, "Nope, I just wanted to smile." And I smile at her, and she grins back at me. And that's it. Right there. That is what it is all about. A shared smile, just for the joy of it. No other reason.

---

[79] https://www.nbcnews.com/better/health/smiling-can-trick-your-brain-happiness-boost-your-health-ncna822591

Here's some tips for learning how to smile more:

- Begin by smiling every time you think of it. If you find you just aren't thinking about it enough, try linking smiling with your triggers alarm 🕐 2, and after you've assessed your feelings, smile (especially if you don't feel like it), and repeat an affirmation in your head.

- Try matching smiles with those around you. If you have kids, smile every time you see them smile. Don't wait until you're feeling happy. Watch them play and when they smile, smile. When they are talking to you, smile. When they do something silly and you're shaking your head in disbelief, try smiling instead! You will notice an immediate effect.

- If you're walking down the street and someone smiles, even if it's not at you, smile.

- Smile when you see someone in your office smile. Even if they are being an arse, even if it is someone on the other side of the room, even if you only see it out of the corner of your eye. The worst that can happen is people will think you are perpetually happy, have a funny joke rolling around in your head, or know something they don't that is keeping you amused. None of these are exactly bad!

- When you've got matching smiles nailed, try smiling when you are angry. This is a tricky one, but so worth it! When your kids are being naughty, when a colleague is being annoying, when a friend is being obnoxious, force yourself to smile. This may mean you have to go hide in the corner to secretly smile, and then go back and address the situation. Or just try smiling to their face.

Smiling when someone is being rude or nasty can often be more effective than getting mad at them. If you smile before speaking, you'll be surprised at how much calmer you are, you'll be less inclined to yell, and generally deal with the situation a whole lot better. I'm still working on this one...

- Be comfortable with smiling. Women statistically smile more than men because it is more socially acceptable. Smiling can often be seen as a form of weakness, minimizing the façade of strength many people wear. But smiling doesn't make you weak; in fact, it takes a strong person to smile in the face of other emotions. Practice smiling throughout your day until it becomes second nature.

- Each morning when you are doing your affirmations in front of the mirror, 🖉 3 smile as you say them. It is easier to make yourself smile when you're in front of a mirror, because you only have to do one, and then you see it. Smiles are contagious, remember. One smile and you'll be able to 'return' the mirror's smile so much easier than if you were just trying to smile without one.

The more you take note of other people's smiles, and start to match them, the more your body and your brain will remember to smile. Not just when you've been prompted by good situations, but all the time. Remember, it is the act of smiling that helps us feel good and lift our moods. You don't have to wait around for something good to happen before you smile.

Need more help smiling? Here's some more things that might help:

- Put yourself in happy situations. Hang out with people you love, and who make you laugh.

- Do activities you really enjoy.

- Watch comedic TV or movies.

- Listen to funny songs or read hilarious books.

- Be mindful ✐4 of your surroundings and find reasons to smile. Find the ladybird in your garden, watch the sun rise, splash in puddles, or dance in the rain.

- Look at pictures of happy moments in your life.

- Imagine a joyful situation in your future.

- Remember a joyful situation from your past.

- Hug a loved one.

- Look up a joke online.

- Attend a comedy show.

- Think of one thing that you are grateful ✐5 for in your life.

There are so many ways to encourage smiling in our day-to-day lives. You just need to start consciously looking for them.

Smiling is amazing. Low mood, stress, and anxiety can all be helped by a simple smile, and they don't cost us a thing. They can make us a kinder, happier person, and make us more attractive to others. What's not to love? Apparently smiling even stimulates the brain's reward system in ways even large amounts of chocolate doesn't, but I don't see why we can't have both chocolate and smiles, just in case...

* * *

RECAP 📌

- Smiling changes your biochemistry and instantly puts you in a more positive state, and bonus - smiling is contagious!

- People who smile are seen as more beautiful, competent, and likeable.

- It's not actually good feelings that make us smile, it's smiles that make us feel good!

- Smiling is the single easiest, cheapest solution to low mood and is available to everyone, everywhere, anytime.

- Low mood, stress, and anxiety can all be helped by a simple smile, and they don't cost us a thing.

ACTION STEPS ✏️

Do now:

- Smile! Big, goofy, teeth showing and eyes crinkling. If you're near a mirror, go smile at yourself in the mirror.

Plan to:

- Smile every time you think about it, especially if you don't feel like it.

- Smile when your trigger alarm goes off.

- Say your morning affirmations while smiling. Preferably in front of a mirror, so your smile is returned!

- Put yourself in happy situations such as meeting with friends or watching, reading and listening to funny material.

- Match smiles with those around you.

Work towards:

- Smiling when you're angry. Use a smile to help you pause, calm down, and address the situation logically.

- Smiling when you're sad. A smile can help lift us out of a wallow and give us a moment of happiness. I find when I smile it helps me find the positives, instead of only seeing the hurt.

LINKED TO

1. Social Butterfly

2. What's Pushing Your Buttons?

3. Say it Like You Mean it

4. Mind Your Mind

5. Great Attitude

GREAT ATTITUDE
♪♫♪ WHAT I GOT — SUBLIME ♪♫♪

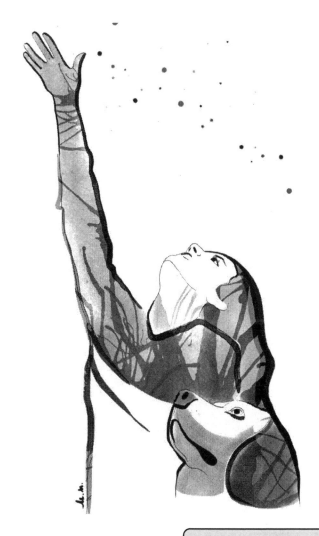

ARTWORK BY MARINA MARKOVA (M.M)

If you were describing your life to someone, what would you tell them? How about your day? Do you talk about all the bad things that happened, or do you focus on the bright moments? Are you an optimist, a pessimist, or a realist?

Turns out it doesn't actually matter. There is new scientific research[80] that shows while you may be genetically predisposed to a positive or negative way of thinking, these traits are not set in stone. They can be changed. This means you can learn to look on the bright side of life, to take how you see a situation and turn it on its head and be happier and more content because of it. 🔗 1

And one of the easiest ways to adopt a more optimistic outlook is to practice gratitude.

Practicing gratitude is an easy exercise that you can do anywhere, anytime. And it is far more valuable than you would think. It helps shift your brain into better ways of thinking, and re-wires it to focus on the good things in life. To change how we see things. Chocolate half left rather than half gone.

😸 The most famous positive psychology intervention is the gratitude exercise. In this exercise people are instructed to jot down three things for which they are grateful. The results show that the gratitude exercise appears to not only boost individual happiness but also buffers people from the deleterious effects of depression.[81]

---

[80] https://link.springer.com/article/10.1007%2Fs11205-009-9559-x
[81] https://www.psychologytoday.com/us/blog/significant-results/201308/whats-so-positive-about-positive-psychology

You see, the more we focus on the bad things in our lives, the tough situations, negative outcomes, and generally crappy things that happens, the more power we give them. There is a story I love that reads:

"One evening an old Cherokee Indian told his grandson about a battle that goes on inside people. He said, 'My son, the battle is between two 'wolves' inside us all.

'One is Evil. It is anger, envy, jealousy, sorrow, regret, greed, arrogance, self-pity, guilt, resentment, inferiority, lies, false pride, superiority, and ego.

'The other is good. It is joy, peace, love, hope, serenity, humility, kindness, benevolence, empathy, generosity, truth, compassion and faith.'

The grandson thought about it for a minute and then asked his grandfather: 'Which wolf wins?'

The old Cherokee simply replied, 'The one you feed.'"

We all have our wolves. The two sides of us that are constantly vying to come out on top. Good vs. Evil if you like. And sadly, we are often so busy feeding the wrong wolf through negative thinking, jealousy, and discontent that it becomes stronger and more powerful, until it is almost impossible for the good wolf to win.

By practicing gratitude, we take that power away. Gratitude not only feeds the good wolf, but the more we're busy feeding our better half, the less time we have to feed the bad. And the longer that good wolf is at the front of our mind, the harder it is for the bad wolf to push him aside.

So how do we practice gratitude? By being mindful 2 of our environment. By seeing all of life, the good and the bad, and then choosing to focus on the good. We can experience bad things, but we don't have to focus on them.◎3 We can think negative thoughts, but we can overwrite them.◎4 We can fail to achieve a goal, but still celebrate how far we've come.◎5

There is always a bright side. A positive slant. A silver lining. It's not necessarily a bad thing to look at life through 'rose tinted glasses.' There is always something you can be grateful for. What good things have happened in your life recently? Some things you could be grateful for right now are:

- Fresh food
- Shelter
- Use of your head, hands, feet, or eyes
- Nature
- Animals
- Music
- Time with friends or family
- Freedom
- Simply being alive
- Education
- The weather, no matter if it is sunny, rainy, snowing or windy. They all have their good points.
- Sunrise or sunset
- Your favourite TV show
- Getting the washing dried
- Having a job that provides for your family
- Completing a chore
- Achieving a goal, or part of one
- Google. I mean seriously, I ask Google so many things! I'm so grateful for Google.
- Clean water
- Friendship

When you practice gratitude, you become happier. Simple.

Life seems to come alive around you, and you wonder how you could possibly have missed all the little things. The deliciously squishy hug from your child, a shared joke, birdsong, the smell of cut grass and fresh bread, new blossoms in spring, and gorgeous leaves in fall. Millions of little things that we overlook while focused on the minutiae of life.

It doesn't always come easy. Gratitude takes practice just like anything else. But it can be life changing!

> ☻ Just two or three weeks of filling out gratitude diaries each evening seems to improve mood, optimistic outlook, and life satisfaction, as well as making you more likely to help others.[82]

This is actually the second time I've written this chapter. I had an awful situation where the program I was using crashed and took 3000 words (about 2 chapters) of my book with it. No backups, no trace. To say I was upset was an understatement. But, I forced myself to find the positives. And this is what I discovered. The more I concentrated on the good aspects of my day, the less upset I became about my lost work.

Don't get me wrong, I was still disappointed, and I reaaally didn't want to re-write what were two of the trickiest chapters in this book, but it wasn't all bad. The day it happened was the last day of a writing week I had been taking with friends. I was tired, and had found the going tough that day, so I had taken time out in the middle of the day for a walk and a swim.

---

[82] https://www.psychologytoday.com/us/blog/the-mindful-self-express/201511/how-gratitude-leads-happier-life

While doing so I met a lovely 74-year-old Irish man and his 16-year-old dog and had a great conversation. I also watched a storm roll in over the ocean which was just gorgeous, spent time with my friends, and wrote a blog post which I didn't lose in the crash. I also didn't lose my previous work - about half the book!

I had so many things to be grateful for! And as I re-write this, I know that it has turned out better the second time around. As many things do. It doesn't matter what happens in life (obviously there are far worse things than losing work), there is always something to be grateful for.

"Gratitude unlocks the fullness of life.
It turns what we have into enough."
-MELODIE BEATTY-

The more we look for silver linings, the easier they are to spot. Sometimes it's difficult to see the one blue patch in a stormy sky, but **even when we struggle to find the positive, we can also learn to appreciate the storm itself, for the way it clears the air, and brings change, and new life.** Everything in life shapes us and strengthens us. The good and the bad.

It's so easy to compare your life to others and see the things you don't have. But practising gratitude helps us look at our lives from a new perspective. It helps us see what we *do* have, and man, we're rich. We have access to clean water, fresh food, a roof over our heads, and clothes on our backs. We are already so much better off than millions of people globally.

'You shall not covet your neighbour's house/wife/donkey' was right up there in the 10 Commandments with 'Don't kill anyone no matter how much they piss you off' (okay, maybe not the exact wording but you get my drift). Comparing yourself to others is such a harmful thing for your mind that it shares space with murdering! We will never be happy as long as we compare ourselves to others and are consumed with desire for (covet) what they have.

Gratitude is all just a matter of perspective. It's choosing to focus on the good in *our* lives instead of comparing ourselves to others or seeing only the bad. It's seeing tough situations as storms to be passed through, and learned from, and life as a series of small events, some of which are wonderful and some of which are not.

Gratitude is not the path we choose as such, but what we choose to focus on, and be grateful for, while on that path.

* * *

RECAP 📌

- One of the easiest ways to adopt a more optimistic outlook is to practice gratitude.

- We all have two wolves inside us. A good wolf, and a bad one. The one we feed with positive or negative thoughts and actions, is the one who wins.

- We practice gratitude by being mindful of our environment, focusing on the good, and being grateful for the things we have.

- Gratitude takes practice just like anything else, but when you practice gratitude you become happier no matter what's going on in your life.

ACTION STEPS ✎.

Do now:

- List everything in your life you have to be grateful for. Don't focus on what you don't have, or what's gone wrong, but instead focus on what has gone right, on what you do have, and on all those wonderful little things around us. List even the little things like hot cups of tea and running water.

- List things you can be thankful for in the future as well, like looking forward to a holiday, a new job, stronger friendships, and keep adding to your list whenever you think of something new.

Plan to:

- Practice gratitude every day, even if you have to remind yourself at first.

- Try an app like 'Mojo' ▶ which encourages you to write 5 things each day you're grateful for. You can add pictures from your phone and link them to dates.

- Take time every night to reflect on something good that happened that day. It doesn't matter how small, find something. While looking for things to be grateful for occasionally is good, it doesn't cement it in your brain like doing so consistently. Practicing gratitude every day is one of the best habits you can get into, and the more you do it, the easier it will become.

- Try writing down your daily 'gratitude' and putting it in a jar. When you are struggling to find something to be thankful for you can pull notes out and reflect on them, remind yourself of all the good things around you. This will encourage you to look at your day with fresh perspective.

Work towards:

- Having gratitude as an automatic response.

- Being able to find the good, even in incredibly bad situations

- Being grateful even for hurtful things in our past that have helped us become who we are today.

- Showing that gratitude to those around you

LINKED TO

1. Happy Happy Joy Joy

2. Mind Your Mind

3. Just Stop It

4. Thinking Too Much About Crap We Shouldn't

5. Aim for the Stars

SAY IT LIKE YOU MEAN IT

♪♫♪ SHUT UP AND DANCE WITH ME — WALK THE MOON ♪♫♪

We cannot always control our thoughts, but we can control our words, and repetition impresses the subconscious, and we are then master of the situation.
-FLORENCE SCOVEL SHINN-

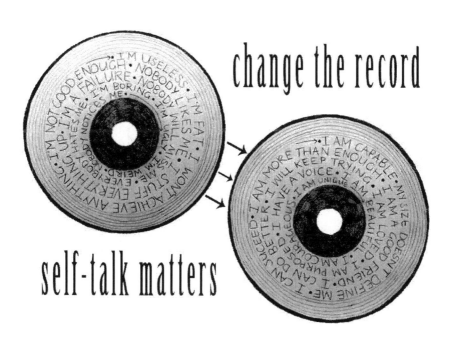

change the record

self-talk matters

ARTWORK BY VANESSA EVETTS

In 'Thinking Too Much About Crap You Shouldn't' 🔗 1, we talked about how negative thoughts are etched into our brains through repetition. Your brain creates easy-access pathways to all those bad thoughts on repeat in your mind, and they become something we think about whether we want to or not.

The key to stopping those negative thoughts is by overwriting them with a mantra, or an affirmation. But what is an affirmation?

An affirmation is simply a short, positive message you tell yourself. They are a conscious thought. Something you can use to recondition your subconscious mind.

When I was growing up, there was a lot of talk about movies and music being laced with subliminal messages. Kids usually found the idea of secret messages quite amusing or even exciting, but adults were a bit more concerned, and with good reason! Subliminal messages go directly to the subconscious mind: the most powerful part of your mind that dictates 95% of your day-to-day thoughts and behaviours.

> ☢ Cognitive neuroscientists reveal that the profoundly more powerful subconscious mind is responsible for 95-99% of our cognitive activity and therefore controls almost all our decisions, actions, emotions, and behaviors.[83]

If your subconscious is on repeat with negative thoughts, then it is incredibly hard to think or feel anything other than negatively. And guess what? 80% of our daily thoughts are negative if we just leave them to their own devices! Why?

---

[83] (Szegedy-Maszak, 2005)
http://www.auburn.edu/~mitrege/ENGL2210/USNWR-mind.html

Because our brains are hardwired to pay more attention to the negative things happening around us, so it can protect us from them. Which was great when we were surrounded by things trying to eat us, but it's not so great now we're at the top of the food chain.

And we have a lot of thoughts! Scientists are still duking it out over accurate figures, but the general consensus is that the average human has anywhere from 12,000-70,000 thoughts a day. That's 8-48 thoughts a minute!

The vast majority of our thoughts (think 95%) are also carried over from one day to the next, meaning they make up the basis of the next day's thoughts. I mean, a caveman's food shortage from yesterday is still going to be an issue today, right? It's not until we actively take control of our thoughts that this figure changes. This is why affirmations are so important!

An affirmation's role is to rewire your mind so that your subconscious thoughts are positive ones. So that the 80% figure changes, and your negative thoughts become less frequent than your positive ones. Affirmations are incredibly powerful and have been proven to make a huge impact on your thoughts and mood.

> ☻ "Researchers looked for and found neural evidence to back up the first two of the hypotheses for why self-affirmation works — the notion that it's beneficial because it's rewarding and pleasurable, and that it works because it acts as a defense mechanism by reminding us of the things in life that we cherish, thereby broadening the foundation of our self-worth."[84]

[84] http://nymag.com/scienceofus/2015/11/why-self-affirmation-works.html#

When you say something often enough you start believing it, and this applies to positive thoughts as well as negative ones. Affirmations help us focus on what we CAN do. They build our self-esteem and self-worth and help us think positively instead of negatively about ourselves, our lives, and our futures.

Affirmations should be short, to the point, and specific to you. Each person will have different things they struggle with in their lives, so it's important to choose your own affirmation - one that really uplifts you and gives you strength.

Here's a list to give you an idea of what you could say with your affirmation.

- I like myself/I love myself
- I am healthy/I will be healthy
- I am incredible
- My mind is clear
- I have energy/I will have energy
- I am well/I will be well
- I am awesome
- I will accomplish my goals today
- I am brave
- I am unique
- I am a good person
- This will pass
- I will get through this
- I will get better
- Life can be good
- Tough times don't last
- I am needed
- I am important
- I am strong
- My past is not my future

When you start using affirmations, begin by using ones that aren't too far away from your point of view. If you hate yourself, start by saying "I like myself," instead of "I love myself." While altering your point of view is important, researchers have found that affirmations too far from what you perceive as true can have a negative effect.

☢ "When positive self-statements strongly conflict with self-perception, there is not mere resistance but a reinforcing of self-perception. People who view themselves as unlovable, for example, find that saying that when they don't really believe it strengthens their own negative view rather than reversing it."[85]

So, take it slowly. Don't jump straight to where you want your head to be at. Take it one step at a time. You have to learn to like yourself before you learn to love yourself. Affirmations are fabulous, but your brain is so conditioned to believing all your negative thoughts that it's not simply going to believe the opposite straight off the bat. But it will if you're consistent.

The best way to use an affirmation is by standing tall and looking into a mirror while speaking out loud. When you see someone (even yourself) saying something, it makes it feel more real. It's easier to believe what's being said. The same is true for smiling into a mirror ⊘ 2.

Pick 1-4 affirmations and repeat them to yourself each morning after cleaning your teeth. Smile. Look yourself in the eye and say it like you believe it. Even if you don't. Remember, an affirmation is about rewiring your brain, creating new, positive

---

[85] https://www.psychologytoday.com/blog/wired-success/201305/do-self-affirmations-work-revisit

pathways for it to follow instead of rehashing negative thoughts.

If you catch yourself having negative thoughts throughout the day, then go straight into your affirmations and say it/them for as long as you need to, to break the cycle of negative thinking.

An affirmation can be used at any time of the day or night to calm, encourage, give you strength, and to help you focus on the positive things in your life. You can use affirmations in conjunction with other hacks such as tapping, @3 smiling, gratefulness, and exercise, @4 and in many different settings, such as:

- In the car

- Before a meeting

- Before an exam

- When you're in a high-stress situation

- When you're angry and trying to calm down

- When you're going for a walk

- In the shower

- When you're struggling to fall asleep or go back to sleep

- As part of your daily routine

- Each time you use the bathroom

- When you're feeling overwhelmed

- Whenever you need a moment of calm

I cannot emphasize enough what a huge difference affirmations can make when used well, especially in conjunction with other mood enhancers such as gratefulness @5 and smiling.

* * *

RECAP 📌

- An affirmation is simply a short, positive message you tell yourself. They are a conscious thought. Something you can use to recondition your subconscious mind.

- 80% of our daily thoughts are negative ones, and the majority of our thoughts are carried over from one day to the next, meaning they make up the basis of that day's thoughts too. An affirmations job is to rewire your mind so your subconscious thoughts are positive ones.

- When you say something often enough you start to believe it, and this applies to positive as well as negative speech.

- Affirmations are incredibly powerful and have been proven to make a huge impact on your thoughts and mood. They build our self-esteem and self-worth, and help us think positively about ourselves, our lives, and our futures.

- The best way to use an affirmation is by standing tall and looking into a mirror while speaking out loud. Take it slowly but be consistent.

- An affirmation can be used at any time of the day or night to calm, encourage, give strength, or to help you focus on the positives in your life.

ACTION STEPS ✎

Do now:

- Write down 10 affirmations that are powerful for you. Keep them short, to the point, and easy to say.

- Go ahead and say them out loud. With oomph!

Plan to:

- Use your affirmations every morning and night after you've cleaned your teeth, and in conjunction with smiling!

- Repeat your affirmations every time you think about them, even if it's only for a few seconds.

- Use your affirmations when you are battling negative emotions.

Work towards:

- Your affirmations becoming your brain's 'go to' subconscious thoughts.

- Being able to overwrite negative thinking, fear, sadness and self-doubt with your affirmations.

LINKED TO 🔗

1. Thinking Too Much About Crap You Shouldn't

2. Smile – Your Face Won't Crack

3. The Weird and the Wonderful

4. Exercise Your Mind

5. Great Attitude

MIND YOUR MIND
♪♫♪ GOOD TO BE ALIVE (HALLELUJAH) — ANDY GRAMMER ♪♫♪

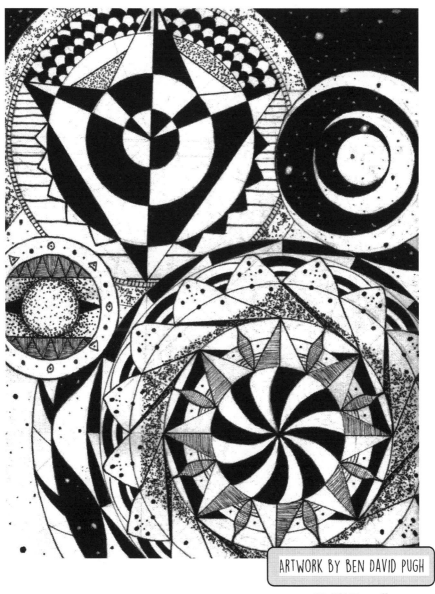

ARTWORK BY BEN DAVID PUGH

In my finance books I speak about mindfulness in relation to money. Being mindful about where and how we spend our money can lead to a greater understanding of its worth and help curtail our spending. But being mindful is not just about money. You can use mindfulness in every area of your life.

Mindfulness is simply being aware of our surroundings and how we interact with them. That's it. Doesn't sound hard, right? And yet most of us go through our day without really registering everything (or anything) that's happening around us.

☢ Psychologist Ulric Neisser found that "your brain is selective in what it sees. Zooming in to focus on one thing always means picking up less information about everything else. That's how we are able to concentrate without the distraction of everything else around us." Our selective brain is how we miss seeing things that are right in front of us. It's also why practicing mindfulness is so important. Not only does it help us see and focus on the good things, it helps us tune out the unhelpful.[86]

There is a fantastic video on YouTube that looks at our awareness ▶. It shows that when we are focusing on only one thing (a tossed ball in this example), that's all our brain sees.

And while you're focused on one part of the story, your brain blocks out whatever else is happening. It's not that it hasn't happened, it's simply that we have missed it. It's like looking at the view through a telescope. The section we are focused on is

---

[86] https://www.scientificamerican.com/article/your-hidden-censor-what-your-mind-will-not-let-you-see/

clear and in detail, but we cannot see anything on the telescope's periphery.

This means we get a distorted view of life. Faulty thinking, negative thoughts, and cultural bias are just some examples of things that can distort our world view ✆ 1. A situation is always neutral, but your thoughts, reactions, and focus on a situation all change what you see and how you react to it.

Learning to live more mindfully means taking notice of the world around us and really seeing it in its entirety. It helps us appreciate and be grateful for the good things in our lives, even the very small ones. The smell of freshly cut grass, the laughter of a small child, the warmth of the sun on your upturned face, these are all things that we take for granted or simply don't notice.

There is more to life than what we usually see. So much more! We need to open our eyes and our minds and really see the world, and our lives. A million different sights, smells, tastes, experiences and occurrences happen all around us that can positively influence our lives, but we have to see them before they can make any impact.

And I don't just mean a glance, a quick 'hey, look at that sunset, now let's get on with the cleaning.' I mean pausing.

Acknowledging the beauty. Breathing. And letting everything else leave our minds other than how glorious that sunset is.

Don't have time? Mindfulness is not about spending hours or even minutes in contemplation. It is surprising how much enjoyment we can gain from being mindful for even a few seconds. Enough time to breath in, and breath out. Anybody can spare a few seconds, especially when you feel more refreshed, positive, and happy for it.

It's so easy to become overwhelmed with everything that's happening in our lives. We complete one task and we're already thinking ahead to the next 10 we have to do! Mindfulness helps us focus on, and enjoy, the here and now. It is present based.

There is a great analogy of living in the present in the book *Too Small to Ignore* by Dr. Wess Stafford. ▶ It is from a speech by an African chief in the 50's, and man, he had a good grasp on mindfulness.

"Time is like a river. It flows along like water, from the future to the present and into the past. But there is a bend in the river. We know the water is coming, but we can't see it or know very much about it, all we know is that it is coming.

The present is now - the days we live today. This is God's gift to us. It is meant to be enjoyed and lived to the fullest. The present will flow by us, of course, and become the past. That is the way of a river, and that is the way of time.

The Frenchmen cannot wait for the future to arrive. They crane their necks to see around the bend in the river. They cannot see it any better than we can, but they try and try. For some reason it is very important for them to know what is coming towards them. They want to know it so badly that they have no respect for the river itself. They thrash their way out into the present in order to see more around the bend.

They stand in the middle of the river, facing upstream, and though the river swirls dangerously around their knees and nearly topples them, they don't care. To them, it seems that the present is only a vantage point to better see around the bend to the future."

All of us have been those Frenchmen at one time or another. Amazing things could be happening around us and we wouldn't even notice. Because we are so focused on seeing around that bend - into the future - that we don't appreciate where we are right now. And that is what mindfulness is all about. Focusing on and enjoying the present moment, regardless of what your past has been like, or what will happen in the future.

Mindfulness can be used for much more than noticing the things happening around you though. It can also be used to explore what's happening *inside* you. Such as keeping tabs on your thoughts and feelings, even those of anger or sadness. Because mindfulness is focused on the present, it gives us the ability to see things as they really are, unlike rumination ⊘ 2, which is focused on the past and tends to warp our perspective. It is not a subconscious action, but a conscious decision. This gives us the ability to explore our emotions without our past experiences or judgements influencing us.

It also means we can use mindfulness to influence how we see and interact with the world. Did you have a bad day? Maybe. Have things gone wrong? Yes. But have things also gone right? When you're mindful, you can see a bad day for what it is. One or two events in an entire day. Several moments that made us feel sad, or angry, or anxious. Not every moment. The events are not cumulative, your whole life is not awful, and there is happiness in every day. And mindfulness helps us find and focus on it.

What would happen if throughout this series of bad events you also focused on the good, however small? When you focus on the small things in your life, as well as the big, you have a much better perspective. You can see that while things definitely go wrong, there were also good things in there too. And that's just life! Life is always going to have its ups and its downs, its good periods and its bad. **Mindfulness is something we can intentionally do to guide our thoughts and our**

responses. This may not sound like much, but it is incredibly important for everybody - especially people with low mood.

You can start learning mindfulness, and influencing your mood for the better, by seeking things out that you already know you enjoy. Little things like sharing a meal with a friend, listening to your favourite song, enjoying the sound of rain on your roof. Having a hot shower, a cup of coffee, or gardening. How many times do you go to drink your coffee and realise that it's already gone? You've been so wrapped up in your thoughts or actions that you've drunk it subconsciously. And right there, you've missed a precious opportunity.

Don't just look, observe. Don't just swallow, taste. Don't just sleep, dream. Don't just think, feel. Don't just exist, live.

A moment of enjoyment has now passed because you weren't focused on the now. This is what it means to be mindful. To really focus on that coffee. Feel the warmth of the mug in your hands, smell the aroma, and taste it as you drink. To actively participate in life, and all of the small things that make it up. Anyone can learn how to transform everyday experiences through mindful awareness.

Enjoying the simple pleasures may not seem monumental, but they can make a huge difference to how we perceive our day, and our lives, and this is what mindfulness is all about. It's not about being forcefully happy or creating situations you can enjoy. It's about focusing on the things in our world that are already happening and giving them the time and attention they deserve. It's about enjoying the moment we're in, and not worrying about the next.

You may start off only noticing one small thing a day, but soon you'll begin seeing more and more things that you simply glossed over in the past. The hug of a child, a pretty garden, the smell of a freshly mown lawn, even just sitting quietly. Being mindful of these moments helps us to exist in the now, instead of focusing on the past or agonising over the future. It also teaches us about what makes us feel good, and gives us things to watch out for, so we can use them to spark happiness again and again.

Mindfulness doesn't compare, because it is only focused on the present. You don't look at the sunset and think, 'I've seen better.' You look at it like it's the first one you've ever seen. It's beautiful on its own terms and in its own right - not in comparison to anything else. Mindfulness doesn't rely on past experiences to create happiness. Instead, it is the sheer ability to focus only on the present moment that makes it so powerful.

How often do you go through your day on auto pilot? Sometimes I drive home and then am shocked that I'm there. I'd spent the whole trip ruminating about the past, or stressing about the future, and hadn't paid any attention to what I was doing.

And I know I'm not alone. I've heard similar stories again and again. If our minds are constantly occupied, we can go through life without ever fully participating, simply going through the motions. Mindfulness stops us hitting the auto-pilot button and gives us back control over what we think about.

Happiness is only ever now. It doesn't have to be complex, in fact it is so often the little things that give us the greatest, and the most lasting joy. And we are missing them, because we are so focused on the future, and our pasts. Stop, breathe, look for the beauty, enjoy the memories, the peace, and the love in your every day and embrace them! Don't let worrying, or planning for your future, ruin any chance of happiness in your present.

Use mindfulness to gain perspective on what's really important in your life and create daily joy instead of looking for future happiness. Be present in your life, and no matter what your day was like, you can ensure your present moment is awesome!

* * *

RECAP ✒

- Mindfulness is something we can intentionally do to guide our thoughts and responses. It is being aware of our surroundings and the small things in life as well as the big, and how we interact with them.

- Mindfulness is not about spending hours in contemplation. We can gain a surprising amount of enjoyment from being mindful for just a few seconds. And anybody can spare a few seconds.

- Mindfulness is all about focusing on and enjoying the present moment, regardless of what your past has been like, or what will happen in the future. To actively participate in life.

- Mindfulness can also be used to explore what's happening inside you. Because it is present focused, it gives us the ability to see things as they really are, unlike rumination, which is focused on the past and tends to warp our perspective.

ACTION STEPS ✎

Do now:

- Write a list of everything, no matter how small, that makes you smile.

- Stop, breathe, and look for one thing right now that is enjoyable. Is the sun shining? Is the moon full? Do you have a child who is alive and well (even though they may be screaming)? Can you make yourself a cup of tea and take a couple of minutes to enjoy it?

Plan to:

- Integrate the things on your list into your daily routine.

- Start practicing mindfulness by setting an hourly alarm. I know, I know, alarms for everything. But they really do work - I promise! When it sounds, stop and take 30 seconds to just breathe and be in the moment. What do you notice about where you are and how you feel right now? What do you notice around you? What is happening in the world? Not just the big things, but the little things. What can you smell? What can you hear?

Work towards:

- Seeing the world around you without having to set an alarm. Focusing on the small, wonderful things that happen every day.

LINKED TO ◎

1. A Positive Spin on Negative Thoughts

2. Thinking Too Much About Crap You Shouldn't

CONCLUSION
♪♫♪ DANCING ON MY OWN — TIESTO REMIX ♪♫♪

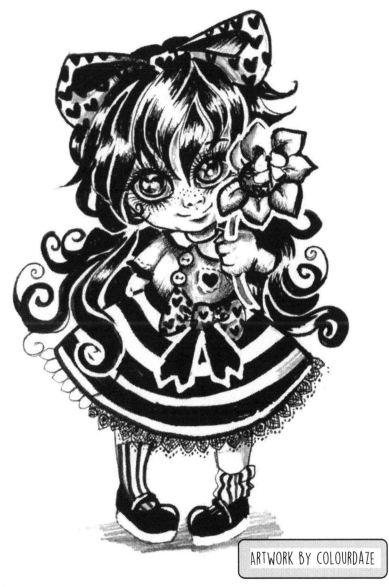

ARTWORK BY COLOURDAZE

Heidi Farrelly • 419

When I visualize my future, I see many things. Family, travel, good friends, and incredible adventures, but the thing that overlies them all is happiness. The kind that other people notice, comment on, and wish for in their lives. The kind that bubbles up inside you and permeates every area of your life. The kind of happiness that you cannot force, but that is an integral part of who you are.

Unfakeable happiness.

Roald Dahl had it right when he wrote:

"If you have good thoughts they will shine out of your face like sunbeams and you will always look lovely."
-ROALD DAHL-

Ever notice how kind people seem more beautiful, even when they are quite plain?

Happiness is no different. When you are truly, genuinely happy, people cannot help but notice. Genuine happiness colours everything you do in life and makes it that little bit more awesome.

Being unfakably happy is my new life goal.

Whether it's implementing a new routine, prioritizing the important things in your life, or learning how to react in difficult situations, every single hack we've talked about in this book helps move you toward one thing: Finding and holding on to genuine happiness.

It will take time to change your perspective on life, see things without distortion, and be grateful for what you have. Be kind to yourself. Your spiral into sadness, apathy, and irritability didn't happen overnight, and neither will your recovery. Take it one step at a time. The great news is you now have all the tools you need to instil and hold onto happiness.

As we've learnt, we are the only ones responsible for our own happiness, and it is up to us to take control of our lives. You, and you alone, get to choose what you think about, each and every day, and are responsible for your own mood. No one else has access to your brain circuitry or can replace your thoughts with their own. They are yours. You control them. And this means you have all the power!

Don't wait around for other people to come to your aid and alleviate your sadness. Your circumstances will not change unless you, and you alone, change your behaviour. Others can support you, but they cannot make changes for you.

If there's one thing I've learnt while researching and trialling hacks to lift mood, it's this: The choices you make, and the things you focus your time and energy on, are the ones that become the most powerful influencers in your life. Yes, people and events in your life can make those choices harder, but you are still the only one who controls your reaction to them, and it is your reactions that shape your life. Not the events themselves.

You see, **the true gift of happiness is that no one can take it away from you.** It is yours to hold, give, share, and enjoy. Being happy doesn't mean that your life is suddenly a bed of roses, it just means that when you are faced with horrible situations, people, and events, you can do so from a much stronger position.

Learning to look at a situation from an alternate perspective, and without the distortion of anger, fear, or sadness can change everything. You are better able to see the positives, learn from situations, and most importantly, move on from them!

But it's not going to happen overnight. Just because you know you should do something, doesn't mean you're going to, right? The ridiculous number of diets half the population has been on is testament to that! So, what's the key to making it all work?

Consistency. Consistency cements things in your brain and helps change single actions into long-lasting habits.

> *"People who consistently make day-to-day decisions that have a positive impact on their life will end up in a vastly different place to those who do the opposite."*[87]

If you do 10 minutes of exercise every day you are far more likely to stick at it, improve on it, and succeed with your goals than if you do an hour's exercise once a week. You don't have to make sweeping changes overnight. In fact, I urge you not to! Instead, start small. Find one hack that calls to you the most, or that you think will be the easiest to implement, and program it into your day.

Use alarms, friends, and family, to encourage and remind you. Litter your home, office, and car with Post-It notes if you have to! Do whatever it takes to implement that one hack into your life. And when you feel like you've got that one nailed, add another one. Several of the hacks go hand in glove, and can

---

[87] http://blog.prymd.com/habits-successful-people/

easily be implemented together, like smiling and affirmations, but just remember it is better to start small and build, than to go all out and then give up.

Be patient with yourself. It didn't take you a week, a month, or even a year, to form the habits and reactions you currently have, and rewiring your brain is not easy.

Be proud of yourself! Consciously working towards positive change in your life is an incredible thing, and one many people never do.

Be kind to yourself. You will not always succeed the first time, or even the second time you try something. But don't give up. Remember, consistency is the key to success.

Above all, be happy. Anger and sadness are both important emotions, and they should never be pushed down or ignored, but they also shouldn't dictate your reactions, or rule your life. When you approach life from a place of happiness and joy, you do so without the distortion of your other emotions. You are able to clearly see situations as they are, and consciously choose your reaction to them. Happiness allows you to be more in control of your life.

After all, you're supposed to be the leading lady in your own life story!

I wish you every success in bringing about positive change in your life, and in defeating sadness, stress, and negative thinking. But above all else, I wish you happiness. Xx

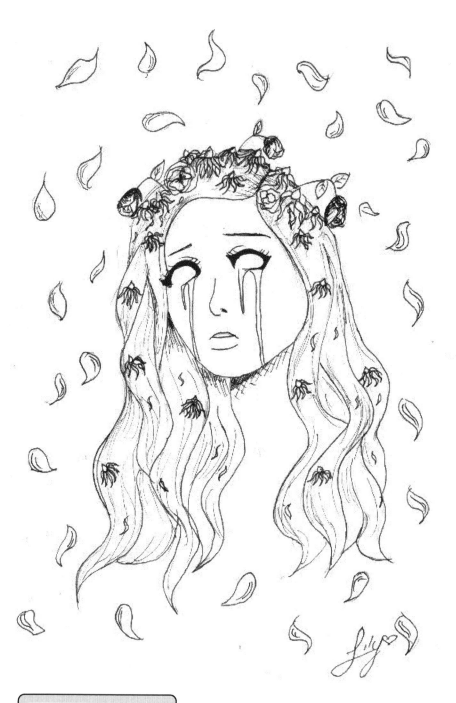

ARTWORK BY LILY BOWDLER

APPENDIX

Symptoms of Depression

Remember that many of these symptoms can also be caused by other health-related issues.

- Difficulty concentrating, remembering details, and making decisions

- Fatigue and decreased energy

- Feelings of guilt, worthlessness, and/or helplessness

- Feelings of hopelessness and/or pessimism

- Insomnia, early-morning wakefulness, or excessive sleeping

- Irritability, restlessness

- Loss of interest in activities or hobbies once pleasurable, including sex

- Overeating or appetite loss

- Persistent aches or pains, headaches, cramps, or digestive problems that do not ease even with treatment

- Persistent sad, anxious, or "empty" feelings

- Thoughts of suicide, suicide attempts, or self-harm

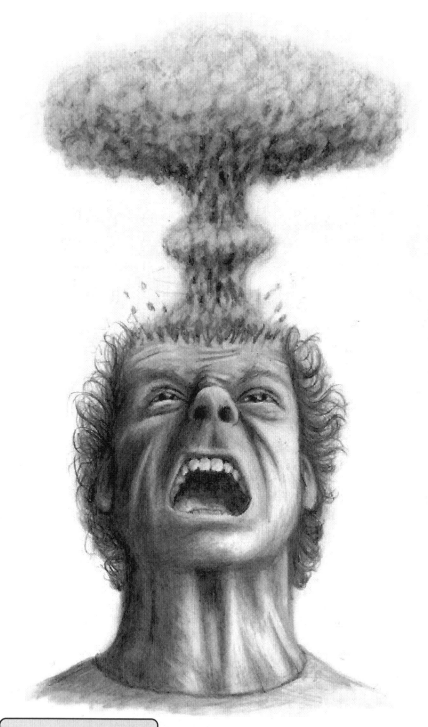

ARTWORK BY CRAIG DAWSON

Websites and Hotlines

Australia - Beyond Blue provides information and support to help everyone in Australia achieve their best possible mental health, whatever their age and wherever they live. www.beyondblue.org.au

Australia - Headspace is a national youth mental health foundation providing early intervention mental health services to 12-25-year old's and their families going through a tough time. 1800 650 890 www.headspace.org.au

Australia - Black Dog Institute is a world leader in the diagnosis, treatment, and prevention of mood disorders such as depression and bipolar disorder. Provides information on symptoms, treatment and prevention. www.blackdoginstitute.org.au

Australia - SANE Australia is a national charity helping all Australians affected by mental illness. 1800 18 7263 www.sane.org

Australia - Relationships Australia is a provider of relationship support services for individuals, families, and communities. 1300 364 277 www.relationships.org.au

Australia - QLife is Australia's first nationally-oriented counselling and referral service for LGBTI people. The project provides nationwide early intervention, peer-supported telephone and Web-based services to diverse people of all ages experiencing poor mental health, psychological distress, social isolation, discrimination, experiences of being mis-gendered and/or other social determinants that impact on their health and wellbeing. 1800 184 527 www.qlife.org.au

Australia - Kids Helpline is a free, private and confidential, telephone and online counselling service specifically for young people aged between 5 and 25. 1800 55 1800 www.kidshelp.com.au

Australia - MensLine Australia is a telephone and online support, information, and referral service, helping men to deal with relationship problems in a practical and effective way. 1300 78 99 78 www.mensline.org.au

Australia - Head to Health is an innovative website that can help you find free and low-cost trusted online and phone mental health resources. www.headtohealth.com.au

Australia - MindSpot Clinic is an online and telephone clinic providing free assessment and treatment services for Australian adults with anxiety or depression. 1800 61 44 34 www.mindspot.org.au

Australia - Carers Australia is a short-term counselling and emotional and psychological support service for carers and their families in each state and territory. 1800 242 636 www.carersaustralia.com.au

Australia - Lifeline is a crisis support and suicide prevention hotline. Call 13 11 14 for help. www.lifeline.org.au

New Zealand - Depression NZ helps to reduce the impact that depression and anxiety have on the lives of New Zealanders by encouraging early recognition and help-seeking. www.depression.org.nz

New Zealand - Mental Health Foundation of New Zealand works towards creating a society free from discrimination, where all people enjoy positive mental health & wellbeing. www.mentalhealth.org.nz

New Zealand - The Lowdown is a website to help young New Zealanders recognise and understand depression or anxiety. www.thelowdown.co.nz

New Zealand - Sparx is an interactive fantasy game that teaches CBT to young people. www.sparx.org.nz

United Kingdom - Mind provides advice and support to empower anyone experiencing a mental health problem. www.mind.org.uk

United Kingdom - Young Minds is the UK's leading charity committed to improving the emotional wellbeing and mental health of children and young people. www.youngminds.org.uk

United Kingdom - SANE runs a national, out-of-hours mental health helpline offering specialist emotional support and information to anyone affected by mental illness. www.sane.org.uk/home

United Kingdom - Friends in Need is a way for people affected by depression to meet online and in their local area. www.friendsinneed.co.uk

United States of America - Anxiety and Depression Association of America is an international non-profit organization dedicated to the prevention, treatment, and cure of anxiety, depressive, obsessive-compulsive, and trauma-related disorders. www.adaa.org

United States of America - Mental Health America is the nation's leading community-based non-profit dedicated to addressing the needs of those living with mental illness. www.mentalhealthamerica.net/conditions/depression

United States of America - National Institute of Mental Health is the lead federal agency for research on mental disorders.
www.nimh.nih.gov/health/topics/depression/index.shtml

United States of America - Reachout delivers peer support and mental health information to youth in a safe and supportive online space. www.us.reachout.com

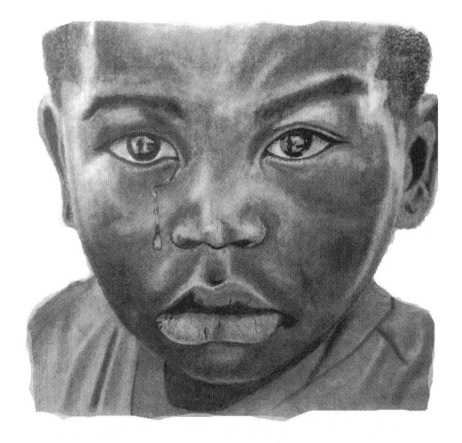

ARTWORK BY LUCKYDAVINCITY

ACKNOWLEDGEMENTS

I owe a huge debt of gratitude to the people around me who keep me grounded and loving life, and who push me to be the best version of myself. A person's support network isn't about who's there for you in the good times, but who's supporting you through the bad, and I'm lucky enough to have some incredible people around me. I hope I can repay you all one day.

Mum, Vanessa, and Michelle, your review work as always has been amazing. Thank you for always making time for me in your busy schedules.

Huge thanks to my friends who gave up their time to read chapters of *Choosing Happy* and provide feedback. It's always great hearing from 'real' people before you hit publish.

To my amazing editor Elaine, who always provides such valuable insights on top of her actual work as an editor. You are awesome.

Sally, the quality of your artwork constantly astounds me. Thank you for putting up with my wild ideas and last-minute changes. I can't imagine my books without your cover art.

To the winners of the #choosinghappyartcomp. You did such an awesome job, and I'm so proud to be showcasing your artwork in my book.

To my long-suffering hubby Clinton and my crazy (like her mother) daughter Molly, thank you for putting up with my eccentricities, my hurricane-like approach to cooking, and my poor housekeeping. And loving me in spite of it all.

And finally, to all the people out there living with an invisible illness. I know what it's like to feel 'less than,' to struggle to get through a day without cracking, and I want you to know you are not alone. You are deserving of love and support. And this too will pass.

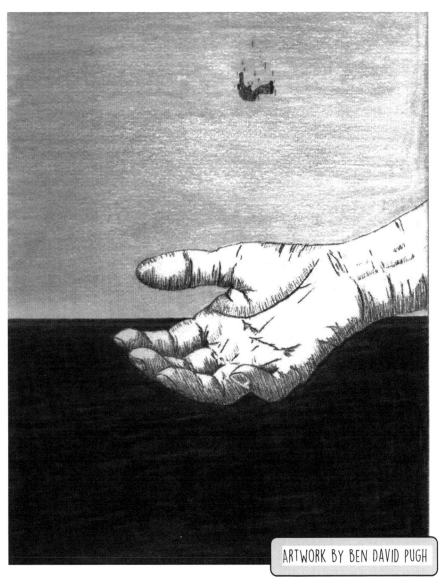

ARTWORK BY BEN DAVID PUGH

ABOUT THE AUTHOR

Heidi lives in sunny Sydney with her husband and daughter, where she loves to swim, rock climb, mountain bike, and cook- all with a hurricane style approach!

She grew up in beautiful New Zealand. You know, that little country at the bottom of the map famous for *Lord of the Rings*, 'Kiwi ingenuity,' adventure, and of course rugby!

Heidi loves to travel and spent 2 ½ years living in and wandering around England and Europe. She tries to explore whenever possible and last year spent 2 weeks trekking through the jungles of Sumatra, where she discovered a new-found hate of leeches.

Heidi is an internationally bestselling author and *Choosing Happy* is her third book. She received widespread media coverage for her previous books *Mortgage Free* and *Brilliant Budgets & Despicable Debt*, appearing live on ABC radio and television's 'The Morning Show,' and headlined top news sources such as *The Daily Mail*, *The NZ Herald*, and *News.com.au*.

Heidi is a top mental health writer for Medium, and her work has also been published by The Mighty, an online community specialising in mental health, invisible illness, disease, and disability.

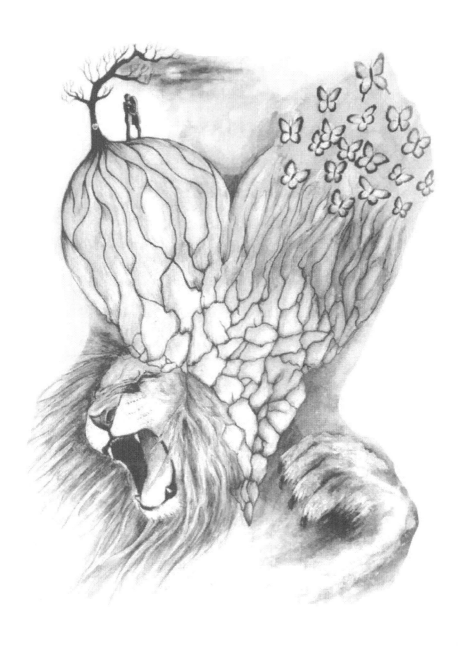

ARTWORK BY CRAIG DAWSON

CONNECT — REVIEW — DOWNLOAD

Heidi loves hearing from her readers! You can connect with her on:

- Medium (@heidifarrelly),

- Facebook (@how2without),

- Instagram (heidifarrellyauthor), and

- Twitter (Heidi2233)

Follow her, leave a comment, or feel free to reshare content from her social media pages that you enjoy or think will benefit others.

If you found this book helpful, please consider leaving a review on Amazon, Goodreads, or any other place that takes your fancy. Reviews help other readers make informed decisions and encourage and support authors.

To download further study links ▶ and bonus materials for this book and her others, please visit the author's website at www.how2without.com. You can also find information on Heidi's previous books here and connect with the artists you've seen within *Choosing Happy*.

I sincerely hope you found *Choosing Happy* to be chock full of goodness. Look out for its companion books - coming soon!

CHAPTER 36

♪♫♪ SHOUT (YOU KNOW YOU MAKE ME WANT TO SHOUT)— OTIS DAY AND THE KNIGHTS ♪♫♪

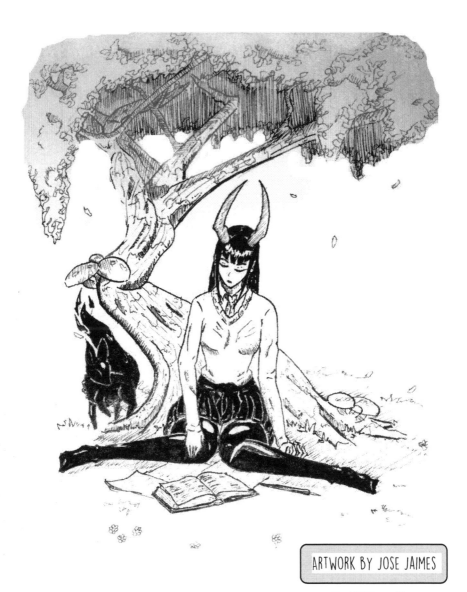

ARTWORK BY JOSE JAIMES

"Hello? Helllllooo? Is anyone there?"

"Well of course there's someone here. You're here. And I'm here."

Jill craned her neck to survey her surroundings, but she couldn't see where the disembodied voice was coming from. And now she'd gone and thought *disembodied*. She shuddered and tried again.

"Who are you? Are you... real?"

"About as real as that quicksand you're standing in" came the altogether-too-cheerful voice.

Jill looked down at the squelching mess tightening around her legs and grimaced.

"About the quicksand. You wouldn't know how I could get out of it, would you?"

"Of course I do! You just spread your wings and fly away".

"Do you see a pair of wings?" Jill questioned indignantly.

"Oh my, you're quite right. How odd."

A twittering laugh echoed through the trees, and finally Jill saw the owner of the voice. A small fantail, perched on a branch above her head, was looking down at her quizzically, its wee head cocked to one side.

"I'm going insane," she whispered, moving her attention from the bird to the grasping goo around her. "And I'm going to be stuck here forever".

A single tear tracked down her cheek, and as if on cue, the stinking sand she was mired in gave a gurgle and sucked her another inch into its grasp.

"Are you insane?" asked the fantail. "I find all the best people are."

Jill tilted her head back and stared at the bird. Why did that phrase sound so familiar? Who knew? Did it really matter anyway?

Above her head, the fantail hopped around on one foot and then the other and began talking again.

"I'm Bob. Get it? Bob." And he did his little bobbing dance again. One foot, then the other, his tail twitching the whole time.

Jill smiled in spite of herself and felt minutely better.

"I don't suppose you know any way out of this quagmire other than flying, do you, Bob?"

Bob paused in his comical dance and thought. "Well, I suppose I might. But first you need to tell me the order of the planets in our solar system."

"What! That is the most ludicrous..." Jill tapered off and sighed as Bob began his dance again, apparently unfazed by her outburst.

Jill grunted. "Ok, fine, why not spend my last moments on Earth telling a talking bird what the names of our planets are."

Jill stared at Bob, blinked and then blinked again. She could have sworn he'd just rolled his eyes at her!

Shaking her head again, Jill straightened up, took a deep breath, and began in her most teacher-y voice. "There are eight planets in total, and in order from the sun they are: Mercury, Venus, Earth, Mars, Jupiter, Saturn, Uranus, and Neptune." Jill was pleasantly surprised to find she didn't even stutter over the order and smiled once again.

"What about Pluto, you forgot Pluto? That was always my favourite planet because it was so little, like me." Bob was hanging upside down and staring at her in a reproving way.

Jill shook her head. "Pluto isn't a planet anymore. Well it is, but they've re-classified it as a dwarf planet." She was getting warmed up to her subject now. She'd always loved space, even when she was little.

"Some fun facts," she continued. "Did you know when it snows on Pluto the snow is red?"

Bob spun right way up again, and shaking all his feathers out said, "No, but that sounds a bit disturbing..."

Jill giggled. "I know, bad image, right? And I have another one for you. Did you know that no human would survive a year on Pluto?"

Bob was dancing again, getting excited. "Let me guess. Let me guess! Bad atmosphere? Man-eating monsters? Scorching sun? Or ooh, ooh, is the blood-red snow actually acid?

Jill shook her head at each guess, her grin widening. "Nope! Although those are some very interesting ideas. Sounds like you've seen 'Pitch Black' one too many times!"

Bob looked a little embarrassed, and Jill gave up questioning how that was even possible.

"Well, what is it then?" he chirped. "Why wouldn't a human survive a year on Pluto?"

"Because you would die of old age before six months was through," she announced triumphantly. "A year on Pluto is equivalent to 248 Earth years."

"You don't say. Well, that wouldn't give you much time to explore, would it!"

Jill shook her head again. "You couldn't stand on Pluto's surface even if you could bypass the ageing problem. It's -378° Fahrenheit, or -228°C if you prefer metric. You'd be an icicle in seconds!"

"Well, I feel very knowledgeable about Pluto now, even if it's not technically one of our planets. Thank you." And Bob inclined his little head to her.

"You're welcome, Bob. Now, would you mind helping me out of this quicksand?"

"But you're already out," Bob chirped, beginning his bobbing dance again.

Jill looked down and found that not only was she out of the quicksand, it had vanished like it had never existed in the first place. She knelt down to prod at the ground. Solid. And dry. And where it had once been, a beautiful little orchid was growing in its place. Jill sat back on her heels and watched as a bee buzzed his way over and began collecting pollen. The sun caressed her back, and in its warmth, she felt so grateful. To be free, to be alive. Standing, she turned her face towards the wood and marvelled that she hadn't noticed its beauty till now.

Bob flew down and landed on her finger like some fairy tale blue jay.

"How?" began Jill. "How did I go from being stuck, to being free without even realising it? And where is the sink-hole?"

"Oh, it's still there, waiting for you."

Jill gave a start and jumped several feet from where she was standing. Bob shook his fuzzy little head. "It doesn't matter how far you go, you'll still find it."

"*I'll* find it? Why on Earth would *I* want to find it?"

"I don't know," chirped Bob. "I've never understood why you humans insist on thinking about things over and over again. You can't fix anything by thinking about it, you know. You have to take action."

"I see. So, you're saying I was just mired in my own thoughts? That it wasn't real? That none of this is real?"

Bob cocked his head. "You're talking to a bird. What do you think?"

Jill smiled and then laughed out loud, surprising herself, and instantly feeling happier.

"So, all the questions about the planets, that was just..."

"A distraction, yes."

Jill shook her head and grinned wryly. "You're good!"

Bob dismissed her praise with a swish of his wing. "Basic psychotherapy," he said. "If you have thoughts you're struggling to get rid of, then stop trying. It's easier to just overwrite them by thinking about something else instead."

"You make it sound so easy," grimaced Jill wryly.

"Wasn't it?"

Jill paused. "You're right. It wasn't that hard. And I bet I could do it again now that I know how."

"Exactly!" Twittered Bob happily.

"Now, I just have one more question." Bob hopped from her right hand to her left and paused his dance long enough to stare at her intently. "How do you remember the order? Of the planets? I always forget things like that!"

Jill chuckled. "I use what's called a Mnemonic. Each word is the first letter of a planet so it's easy to remember. **M**y **V**ery **E**ducated **M**other **J**ust **S**erved **U**s **N**oodles".

"Oh, that's very clever. But I don't like noodles," said Bob, flying back to his branch. "They remind me too much of worms."

"You don't like worms?" queried Jill. "What kind of a bird are you?"

But Bob was gone, leaving Jill to enjoy the beautiful morning. And it was beautiful, now that she'd begun to pay attention. The sun was shining, she'd learnt a new trick for overcoming her nagging, negative thoughts, and she'd rediscovered a subject she loved. She smiled, and a delicious feeling of well-being shot through her as she began to make her way along the path.

Happy.

Made in the USA
San Bernardino,
CA

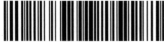
59006969R00250